Sally Farmiloe - Nei
2005. —

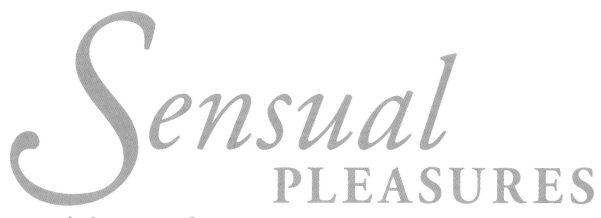

Sensual
PLEASURES
and the ART of MORPHING into a HEALTH GODDESS

Sally Farmiloe-Neville

BOOK GUILD
PUBLISHING

The Book Guild Ltd
25 High Street
Lewes, East Sussex
BN7 2LU
www.bookguild.co.uk

and

Delancey Press Ltd
23 Berkeley Square
London
W1J 6HE
www.delanceypress.com

First published 2005

Edited by Tatiana von Saxe
Designed and produced by Mirabai Ltd
Printed and bound by W S Bookwell

ISBN 1 85776 989 9
      978 1 85776 9890

For my family … in both realms

ACKNOWLEDGEMENTS

I would like to thank the following, without whom this book would not have been written:

TATIANA VON SAXE, my wonderful publisher, editor and friend who dreamed up the idea and worked her butt off to get *Sensual Pleasures and the Art of Morphing into a Health Goddess* published on time.

CAROL BISS, my dynamic co-publisher who came up with the title and who supported and flattered me at all times.

All of our outstanding CONTRIBUTORS who cheerfully gave me so much of their precious time and valuable advice for no remuneration and who made this book so comprehensive.

My patient housemates JEREMY, JADE and KAT who respected a closed study door and knew that when I was in literary mode I was not likely to be a domestic goddess as well!

Contents

PREFACE   viii

Section one   TASTE

1   FOOD   1
Food tips   1
The banana – its many uses   2
Weight and dieting tips   3
Weight and hypnosis   4
Kinesiology   6
Three course no wheat no dairy menu   7
Novelli's Vegetarian Pipérade   8
Alternatives to diet   9
Eating "up" the evolutionary scale   9
Food combining   11

2   DRINK   12
Water, soft drinks and juice   12
Dental advice   13
Looking after your teeth   13
Tooth loss   14
Alcoholic drinks   14
Alcohol and hypnotherapy   15
Alcohol dependency/addiction   15

3   SMOKING, DRUGS, MEDICATION,
VITAMINS ET AL.   16

4   EAT YOUSELF HEALTHY: DISEASE
PREVENTION PLUS ANTI-AGEING,
MENOPAUSE AND HORMONES   18
Cholesterol   18
Coronary heart disease   19
Strokes   20
Diabetes   20
Prevent diabetes, prevent ageing   21
Anti-ageing   22
The menopause   22
The menopause and HRT   23

5   FOOD FOR THOUGHT: THE BRAIN,
THE MIND, THE SOUL   27
Fish   27
Coffee   27
Three course fish menu   28
Integrative Psychotherapy   29
Depression   29

6   CELLULITE AND FATTY
TISSUES AND ISSUES   30
So what exactly is cellulite anyway   30
Cellulite treatments   31
Mesotherapy   31
Endermologie   31
Meso-mesh   32
Tri-Active   33
Lipostabil   33

7   EXERCISE   34
Exercise to keep your body young and fit   35
What is aerobic exercise?   36
Ballroom dancing   36
Belly dancing   36
Yoga   38
Tennis   39
Swimming and water sports   39
Skiing and snowboarding   40
Health & fitness clubs   40
Some fitness and nutrition myths   40
Natural secrets   41
The natural way   42
Pilates   43
Back pain   43
Posture   45
Feldenkrais method – pains and injuries   46
Foot care   48

Section two  SMELL

8   ARE YOU FRAGRANT?   49
    Products   49

9   SMELL AND FOOD AND THINGS   51
    Three course fragrant menu   52

Section three 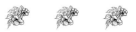 SIGHT

10   BEAUTY: MAKE-UP   53
     Face products   53
     Colour conscious   54
     Dark skin   55
     Black beauty   55
     Asian skin   56
     Make-up tips   57
     Hair products   58

11   BEAUTY: SKIN CARE   59
     Skin care products   59
     Dermatologists   60
     Skin conditions   61
     Skin care   63
     Natural care   64

12   BEAUTY TREATMENTS: FACE,
     HAIR AND BODY   66
     What is available   66
     Home beauty treatments   67
     Hair removal   69
     Hair colour and styling   70
     Hair extensions   70
     Non-surgical face lift   71
     Waxing   71
     Nails   71
     Wigs   72
     Spas   72
     Medispa treatments   72
     More spas   74

13   THE SUN AND ITS EFFECTS
     AND FAKE TANS   76
     Products   76
     Tanning   77
     Fake tanning products   78

14   BEAUTY: THE SERIOUS STUFF   79
     Botox   79
     Evolence   80
     Aquamid   81
     Cutera lasers   82
     Cynosure lasers   82
     Anti-ageing   82
     Intense Pulsed Light Treatment   83
     Titan procedure   83

15   ALTERNATIVE HEALTH
     TREATMENTS   84
     Colonic irrigation   84

16   BEAUTY: EVEN MORE SERIOUS STUFF   87
     A short history of face lifting   88
     Isolagen and Thread Lifting procedures   89
     Cosmetic surgery   90
     Advice on cosmetic surgery   91
     Photo imaging   92

17   SIGHT: LOOKING AFTER YOUR EYES
     AND KEEPING THEM HEALTHY   93
     Eye care   93
     Laser eye surgery   93
     Eyes and eye care   94
     A patient's experience with Accuvision   94
     Wavefront guided LASIK at Accuvision   95

18   THE SENSUAL PLEASURES OF SIGHT   96
     Things of beauty   96
     Permanent make-up   96
     Colour Me Confident   98
     What to wear   99
     Body shapes   99
     Fashion   99
     Accessories   100
     Stylists   101
     Three course menu recipes – presentation   102

Section four  HEARING AND SOUND

19 EAR CARE 104
Remedies and methods 104

20 SOUND AND MUSIC 105
Favourite music 105
Meditation 106
Snoring 108
Insomnia 108

21 VOICES 110
Educating the voice 110
Voice – does it matter? 111

Section five TOUCH

22 STROKING AND MASSAGE 112
What good is a massage? 112
Neuro-muscular massage 113
Sports massage 113

23 TOUCHY FEELY 114

**24 LOVE AND ROMANCE AND
A BIT OF SEX** 115
Suggested menu for love 115

**25 GYNAECOLOGY AND SEX:
THE SERIOUS STUFF** 117
Gynaecological and obstetric advice 117
Sexually transmitted diseases 120
Sex addiction 122

26 SEX: THE FUN STUFF 124
Exercises and techniques 124

EPILOGUE 125

LIST OF CONTRIBUTORS 126

INDEX 128

Preface

THIS book is for women and girls of all ages. It is my true belief that you are never too young to start looking after your health, not to mention your looks, and never too old to maintain them.

We all need sensual pleasures in our lives. Sensual pleasures put the "joie" into "vivre". Or, as the romantic *Phantom of The Opera* advised, "exercise your senses…".

To really enjoy life and to get the most out of it, it is important to be truly healthy. We cannot all be love goddesses, sex goddesses or beauty goddesses but we can all be Health Goddesses.

Taste

I
FOOD

Food is the big one in most women's lives for one reason or another and we have to address this ticklish subject first and foremost.

Food tips

"You are what you eat." This is not a cliché, it is one hundred percent true. Whether you suffer, God forbid, from malnutrition, anorexia, bulimia or binge eating, you will never achieve perfect health until you sort out your food intake. *"My body is my temple"*, some people say. But would you treat it so badly if it really was your temple? There has to be a balance nutritionally.

If you are someone who watches her weight, you will know that you can easily put on pounds in one binge day and take it off again in one restrained one. We all enjoy the really sensual pleasure of eating delicious yummy foods but we hate what some foods do to our looks. Not only do those double chocolate chip cookies add inches *("a moment on the lips, a lifetime on the hips")* they are also bad for the skin and the teeth.

The famous skinny beauties, including THE DUCHESS OF WINDSOR and JACQUELINE KENNEDY ONASSIS, who told us we could never be too rich or too thin were wrong on the second count. You absolutely *can* be too thin, especially as you get older and your skin loses elasticity. Whether you tend to be too big or too small, you need to find a way of eating that suits you. Yo yo dieting is the worst thing you can do to your body because if you are alternately putting on and taking off weight, you are stretching your skin and its natural elasticity will not last forever. *Moderation* is the key if you

tend to put on weight. Do not deny yourself foody treats, your sensual pleasures of taste, but make them small and infrequent. Nobody can stay on a constant diet, it is just too-too boring: eat sensibly most of the time with the odd tasty delight to satisfy your taste buds.

For those of you who *do* have to watch your weight you may become obsessive about food and this is a slippery slope. You need to take your mind off the dreaded subject of food and give yourself other treats when you feel hungry. For instance if your husband or lover is not immediately to hand, so to speak, you can surprise him with a sexy phone call at the office (but beware the BRIDGET JONES speakerphone possibility!). That should take your mind off the unhealthy sticky donut you were contemplating. Or, if your loved one is out or in conference, how about a good old gossip with a girlfriend? Or treat yourself to watching a daytime soap or a video or even a chapter of the latest juicy novel? Get on the Internet and e-mail your mates; the latest funny Net joke will do it as long as it is not about food. If necessary nip off to HARRODS, or your local de luxe store, and salivate at other things besides food (stay away from the food hall!). Anything to stave off those hunger pangs until it is time for a proper (healthy, nutritional) meal. I promise you, this will work, you just need to put your tea and "elevenses" times aside for something other than food. Once you stop obsessing about food you will feel much less hungry.

JANE FONDA, one of the most beautiful and well-preserved bodies in the fitness business, said she only gained control of her weight once she stopped thinking about it the whole time. So put the scales away, except for a weekly check up to keep an eye on things and enjoy your food in moderation. If you do go mad every now and then, you will just have to eat less the next day. The best advice I can give you vis a vis food is to *eat slowly*: chew each mouthful ten times and you will be helping your digestion as well as your waist line.

There are so many good diet foods around nowadays, it is not really so difficult to lose or maintain weight. The best meal replacements, which are ideal for quick meals, are the famous SLIM-FAST shakes, bars and soups beloved of VICTORIA BECKHAM and BOOTS' SHAPERS who do a similar range. The only problem with these sorts of diet foods is that they are not exactly fresh food so they will not be helpful to you nutritionally or if you have a tendency towards cellulite – but we will come to that shortly. On the subject of diet foods, do read the labels carefully: some products may be low-fat or indeed no-fat, but they are full of sugar, salt and preservatives. Sugar and salt are fattening in large quantities and preservatives are not good for your health or your cellulite, should you have any. There is no replacement for fresh food so try not to eat diet foods for too long if you want to be truly healthy. Sometimes it is better to be a slightly bigger size (which is often more appealing to men anyway) with glowing skin, shining hair and a good digestion than skinny as a rail but looking and feeling unhealthy.

If you are looking for a really healthy lactose free dietary supplement with no artificial sweeteners, try WHEY TO GO whey protein powder. This product, available from speciality health food stores, is ideal not just for losing weight but for women with serious food intolerances. One aficionada of "WHEY TO GO" is healthy beauty PRINCESS KATARINA OF YUGOSLAVIA (aka MRS DESMOND DA SILVA) who swears by it.

PRINCE CHARLES and LIZ HURLEY have admitted that they only eat one meal a day to keep their weight down. This is fine if you are a lioness but human bodies thrive on little and often. Three or four small meals a day are much better for your digestion and remember, if you suffer, for instance, from excessive heartburn caused by protracted periods with no food in your stomach, your skin, your eyes and your general well-being will all be adversely affected. If you must only eat one meal a day, do put something soothing into your poor tum during the day: milky drinks are good and nibbling on raw carrots, celery and apples will keep you going until dinner time without piling on the calories.

In fact do take another look at fruit as an alternative sweet taste to that naughty chocolate we all love so much,

not to mention all the chocolate flavoured diet bars and drinks. We now know that we are supposed to eat five portions of fresh fruit or vegetables a day to ward off cancer and it is definitely a sensual pleasure to eat cherries, grapes, mangoes and other exotic fruits which are now all cheaply and cheerfully available in our local markets. Try to eat fresh fruit at the end of a meal instead of a sweet sickly pud – or "dessert" as would-be posh nosheries like to call it! (Unless, of course, you have digestive problems and find that eating fruit with other food churns up your stomach and causes unattractive flatulence in which case you should always eat your fruit separately.)

The banana – its many uses

Fruit eaten by itself can make a satisfying whole meal and will give plenty of instant energy. Even the humble banana has now reached an elevated position in our daily diets. Opposite is a fascinating report on this super-convenient fresh fruit sent to me by HOT GOSSIP UK's Canadian fitness correspondent, WILLIAM DRYSDALE.

Slippery banana skins have long been a cartoon joke but did you know the banana skin has another use entirely? Over to GEORGINA BRUNI, my esteemed Editor In Chief at popular (Internet and hard copy) magazine HOT GOSSIP UK, founder of Knightsbridge social club, CLUB 2000 and PR lady extraordinaire.

INSTANT FACE LIFT

This is a fabulous recipe for an instant face lift, which works a dream if you have a hangover or are not feeling well and have to go out socialising.

One banana

1 Cleanse face and neck. Rinse with cold water.
2 Take the skin of a banana and using the inner peel (the white part) gently rub it into the face and neck.
3 Leave it for approximately **ten** minutes or until it tightens and turns brown.
4 Rinse with warm water, then cold.
5 Your face will feel and look terrific. The skin will feel smooth and tight – and you can eat the banana…

BANANA FACTS THAT MAY SURPRISE YOU

After reading this, you'll never look at a banana in the same way again!
Containing three natural sugars – sucrose, fructose and glucose combined with fibre – a banana gives an instant, sustained and substantial boost of energy. Research has proven that just two bananas provide enough energy for a strenuous 90–minute workout. No wonder the banana is the number one fruit with the world's leading athletes.

But energy isn't the only way a banana can help us keep fit. It can also help overcome or prevent a substantial number of illnesses and conditions, making it a must to add to our daily diet.

Depression: According to a recent survey undertaken by MIND amongst people suffering from depression, many felt much better after eating a banana. This is because bananas contain tryptophan, a type of protein that the body converts into serotonin, known to make you relax, improve your mood and generally make you feel happier.

Anaemia: High in iron, bananas can stimulate the production of haemoglobin in the blood and so help in cases of anaemia.

Blood pressure: This unique tropical fruit is extremely high in potassium yet low in salt, making it perfect to beat blood pressure. The US Food and Drug Administration have just allowed the banana industry to make official claims for the fruit's ability to reduce the risk of high blood pressure and stroke.

Brain power: 200 students at a Twickenham (Middlesex) school were helped through their exams this year by eating bananas at breakfast, break and lunch in a bid to boost their brain power. Research has shown that the potassium-packing fruit can assist learning by making pupils more alert.

Constipation: High in fibre, including bananas in the diet can help restore normal bowel action, helping to overcome the problem without resorting to laxatives.

Hangovers: One of the quickest ways of curing a hangover is to make a banana milkshake, sweetened with honey. The banana calms the stomach and, with the help of the honey, builds up depleted blood sugar levels, while the milk soothes and re-hydrates your system.

Heartburn: Bananas have a natural antacid effect in the body, so if you suffer from heartburn try eating a banana for soothing relief.

Mosquito bites: Before reaching for the insect bite cream, try rubbing the affected area with the inside of a banana skin. Many people find it amazingly successful at reducing swelling and irritation.

Nerves: Bananas are high in B vitamins that help calm the nervous system.
Overweight and at work? Studies at the Institute of Psychology in Austria found pressure at work leads to gorging on comfort food like chocolate and crisps. Looking at 5,000 hospital patients, researchers found the most obese were more likely to be in high-pressure jobs. The report concluded that, to avoid panic-induced food cravings, we need to control our blood sugar levels by snacking on high carbohydrate foods every two hours to keep levels steady.

Ulcers: The banana is used as the dietary food against intestinal disorders because of its soft texture and smoothness. It is the only raw fruit that can be eaten without distress in over-chronicler cases. It also neutralises over-acidity and reduces irritation by coating the lining of the stomach.

Temperature control: Many other cultures see bananas as a "cooling" fruit that can lower both the physical and emotional temperature of expectant mothers. In Thailand, for example, pregnant women eat bananas to ensure their baby is born with a cool temperature.

Seasonal affective disorder (sad): Bananas can help SAD sufferers because they contain the natural mood enhancer, tryptophan.

Stress: Potassium is a vital mineral, which helps normalise the heartbeat, sends oxygen to the brain and regulates your body's water balance. When we are stressed, our metabolic rate rises, thereby reducing our potassium levels. These can be rebalanced with the help of a high-potassium banana snack.

Strokes: According to research in *The New England Journal of Medicine*, eating bananas as part of a regular diet can cut the risk of having a stroke by as much as 40%.

Warts: Those keen on natural alternatives swear that if you want to kill off a wart, take a piece of banana skin and place it on the wart, with the yellow side out. Carefully hold the skin in place with a plaster or surgical tape!

So, a banana really is a natural remedy for many ills. When you compare it to an apple, it has four times the protein, twice the carbohydrate, three times the phosphorus, five times the vitamin A and iron, and twice the other vitamins and minerals. It is also rich in potassium and is one of the best value foods around. So maybe it is time to change that well-known phrase so that we say, "A banana a days keeps the doctor away!"

Weight and dieting tips

Women cannot live on bananas alone so what else should we eat to keep us healthy? To go organic or not to go organic, this is the question.

Hypnotherapist VALERIE AUSTIN (118 Piccadilly, London W1, phone 020 7702 4900, www.valerieaustin.com), pioneer of the world-famous AUSTIN TECHNIQUE is also an authority on nutrition and has this to say:
"Think of organic as real food and anything else as tampered with or synthetic.

It is important to read all labels carefully. You will see the amount of salt and sugar that is in the food – acquaint yourself with any names you do not understand. There are many food ingredients and additives that can create emotional stress and make anxiety that much worse.

Buy vegetables from reputable organic shops whenever possible rather than supermarkets – you will notice the difference. The shape will be different with no bright artificial colours.

I have joined the many frustrated people that have bought a bread machine so that I know what I am eating and I am surprised how easy it is.

Even organic bread can have far too much salt and is made with vegetable or palm oil. Vegetable oil is called 'heart attack on a plate' in the United States. Look for bread made with olive oil but I can assure you it won't be easy. It has to do with manufacturers using cheap oil to cut the price and using salt and sugar as preservatives to get that long, long shelf-life.

A friend of mine said that if she were to eat like I suggest she would be shopping every other day. I asked her to remember that this was normal when people were not dying all over the place and no one had heard of dodgy knees and hip replacements. The only reason that we can buy for a whole month is 'shelf-life'.

This 'shelf-life' is what is killing us. I always remember the saying 'there are no free lunches'. There certainly aren't when dealing with food. Longer shelf-life probably equals shorter life."

Many people think that organic food is too expensive but my feeling is that you will save money on medications, especially cold and flu remedies, if you eat more healthily, i.e. go organic. Above all try to eat as much fresh food as possible and do not drown nice healthy salads in dodgy salad dressings: NEWMAN'S OWN, for instance, is made with all natural ingredients and therefore is quite healthy although olive oil and vinegar or fresh lemon juice by themselves have got to be the safest option.

Back on the weight loss business, if you really have a problem in shifting those pounds and inches, why not try hypnotherapy? If you have the time and the money it is always more relaxing to be hypnotised by a trained practitioner such as VALERIE. However you can actually hypnotise yourself! Here, in an excerpt from her best selling book, *Slim While You Sleep*, VALERIE talks you through her self-hypnosis technique and teaches you how to "suggest yourself slim":

WEIGHT & HYPNOSIS

Induction to hypnosis to be played on a tape or read by a trusted friend or relation and follow it with the suggestion you require, for example weight, insomnia, etc.

Progressive Induction

I want you to imagine that you're checking your body to ensure you become totally relaxed… As your muscles relax, just let your mind relax also… Begin with your feet… Feel your toes… stretch them, feel the texture of (the floor, your shoes/socks) against your feet… and relax them… Begin to tighten your calves… now relax them… let that relaxation spread past your ankles up your calves to the back of the knees… Feel those muscles easing… resting… comfortably… Now your thighs, pull them tight… be aware of those long muscles tensing – now relax those muscles, feel them lengthening and resting comfortably… Feel your legs as they sink even deeper into the cushions as you relax even more… if you've done this properly your legs seem to sink deeper into the cushions of the (chair/bed)… as you allow yourself to relax even deeper… Notice

how regular and rhythmic your breathing has become… Now your stomach muscles, pull them in gently… now let them expand and relax comfortably.

Your shoulders and back muscles… flex them… feel them pull across your back as you relax… and notice how your spine sinks deeper into your chair. As you relax even more deeply.

Notice how easy and regular your breathing has become… Now your fingertips and fingers… clench them… feel that tension… Now relax them… and allow the relaxation to spread up your arms to your neck… Make sure your neck is comfortable with your head in an easy position.

Your face muscles are flat and stretch comfortably across your face… Squeeze up your face… and feel the tension… now relax those muscles and feel them lengthening… and softening… relaxing more than ever before.

You can now feel the air temperature against your skin… It feels smooth and comfortable… Now you can allow the relaxation to spread to your scalp… knowing that you are relaxed… from the top of your head… to the tip of your toes.

In a moment I will ask you to open your eyes and find an imaginary spot on the ceiling… Your job is to fix your eyes on that spot and focus on that spot and not let your eyes wander… Open your eyes now (when they open their eyes you look up at the ceiling yourself which encourages them in case they are not sure).

As your eyes are [fixed] on that spot I will ask you to count backwards… from 500 rhythmically and silently… and while you are doing that I will be talking to you… but you need not pay any special attention to what I say… but you will hear me when I tell you to stop counting… so start counting now.

As you keep looking at that spot you realise that the only part of your body that is working hard is your eyes. They may become watery or dry so let them blink as often as they like. (As soon as you see a blink of their eyes remark:) the more your eyes blink the more tired your eyes become… and soon they will want to close and rest like the rest of your body.

If their eyes are still open just say "Just close your eyes". If the eyes are still open say in a louder voice "Just close your eyes".

You can stop counting now. Your body is now loose and limp… and heavy… and relaxed. Now you're so deeply relaxed… you find it easy to focus your attention and imagine things very clearly… and I want you to imagine that you are standing on a balcony which has steps leading down to a beautiful garden… surrounded with lovely trees… making sure the garden is private… secluded… and peaceful… The green lawn

has clusters of beautiful flowers… Do you see the flowers?… (Wait for response) If you look more closely you will notice that there are five steps leading down to a lower terrace and five more steps to the lawn itself.

In a moment I want you to walk down the first set of steps and you will become more and more relaxed…

Now in your mind's eye I want you to put your foot on the first step… and as you do you find yourself becoming beautifully and deeply relaxed… The second step… even more relaxed… The third step even deeper relaxed… The fourth step… deeper still… The fifth step even deeper still… As you are standing at the bottom of the steps you notice a large stone vase to one side filled with beautiful flowers. What colour are the flowers? (Wait for response)

Now I want you to walk down the next five steps to the garden itself… and with each step you will become even more

deeply relaxed… so let's begin. (Repeat above for the second set of steps) When you reach the bottom steps you'll see a comfortable garden bench. What colour is the bench? (Wait for response)

In a moment I will ask you to walk over to that bench… and when you get there I will ask you to sit down… and when you sit down you will be even more deeply relaxed than you are right now… So let's begin… it's not far (leave three seconds). Now sit down… take a deep breath… and as you breathe out… you can become beautifully and deeply relaxed. Whenever I work with you again and I say the words "and sleep" you will go quickly and easily into even deeper relaxation.

Follow this with a suggestion. You can use those below to help you get started, adding words that are more suitable to you.

Weight Control Suggestions (1)

Your weight is reducing, and you achieve and maintain your desired weight.

You are happy, secure and confident in the knowledge that you eat more rationally, eating lower calorie, healthier foods. You

discover to your pleasure, that you are fully satisfied on smaller amounts of food.

Your metabolism works at an increased speed, burning up the small amounts of food that you enjoy eating and ensuring that your body stays firm and slim.

You are thrilled with your reflection in the mirror. You are amazed at how much healthier and more energetic you feel and how much more you enjoy life.

You radiate vitality and you are proud of your new healthy body.

Weight Control Suggestions (2)

Because you want to lose weight and become healthier and fitter, each day you eat the food that you know is good for you. You enjoy healthy food. You no longer crave high calorie rich foods and enjoy eating low calorie healthy foods. Your subconscious knows which foods are good for you and allows you to lose weight at the rate suitable for your body. Day by day you eat only when you are physically hungry

and you eat and want only those foods that are good for your body. You always sit down when you eat and enjoy drinking water. You find it very cool and refreshing and you like the taste. You find yourself much more thirsty than you formerly were. Your stomach is smaller and getting smaller with every day that passes. You visualise your stomach as small.

You always leave food on your plate and day by day you are enjoying a new eating

habit. You only think of the bite that is in your mouth and because you think only of the bite that is in your mouth, you enjoy the taste of it much more. Your taste buds become more sensitive and you get much more satisfaction from each bite. You eat more slowly, you eat much less, but you enjoy it more. You are looking better and you are feeling better. You feel good about yourself.

If you are too thin or are a recovering anorexic or bulimic, your problem is altogether more fun: you can enjoy the sensual pleasure of eating yourself bigger. Remember, as you age you will actually look younger if you are carrying a bit more weight so mature gals can also afford to eat a bit more. If you really have no appetite, you will need to tempt yourself with yummy food and you can eat your nanas with lashings of fresh cream and honey (so much better for the health and teeth than sugar). However fatty foods alone will not put on the weight and make you healthy, you will need to follow the same well balanced protein, carbohydrate and fat diet as your larger sisters – just more of it.

Ageless beauty and famous film star SOPHIA LOREN reckons she has always had to eat up to keep her figure luscious and recommends pasta to build up the curves. This is fine in moderation but too much wheat is never healthy and you must eat your regular quota of fresh food, particularly vegetables and fruit, as well. Raw vegetables are particularly healthy and, in her wonderful book *Sophia Loren's Recipes and Memories* (published by Gremese and available from W.H. Smith) the sultry star features a hot spaghetti with a cold "sauce" of uncooked tomatoes, onions, green olives, etc. in olive oil which is as refreshing as it is healthy in summer. Try it, ladies.

Congratulations if you are pregnant and eating for two. Now your body is not just your temple but your baby's as well so do still follow a balanced diet and try to resist too many ghastly cravings. Pregnancy is not an excuse to throw caution to the wind and go mad on the eating front: you will only have to lose it all again after the birth. However if you suffer from the dreaded "morning sickness" during pregnancy this is the one time when I recommend drinking hot, sweet tea with lots of sugar and carbonated drinks such as (non-diet) COCA-COLA as it really seems to settle a nauseous stomach. (In fact these drinks work pretty well for nausea and sickness of any sort while burned toast is the safest thing to eat for sickness. Obviously if you often feel sick and are not pregnant you should see your doctor immediately.)

Once you have had your sprog and are breast feeding (a must for a healthy baba for at least three months) it is positively desirable to eat lots of carbs to build up baby as well as yourself. Your pregnancy weight should fall off quickly if you are breast feeding (and did not gain too much while preggers) but you will have to resume your usual diet once you stop so do not get too used to your apple crumble and cream!

If you want to know more about keeping yourself fit (not fat) and healthy during and after pregnancy, do invest in my video, *Regain Your Figure: Easy Exercises For Expectant and New Mothers*: £14.99 from Farmingham Productions, 12 Tilton Street London SW6 7LP, phone 020 7381 5735, e-mail farminghamprods@aol.com). Just thought I would mention that!

We are always being told that we all eat too much wheat and dairy products. We probably do so for reasons of convenience: it is so easy to eat sarnies, cheese, pasta, cereal with milk, etc., not to mention drinking lots of milky drinks. If you feel there is a predominance of wheat and dairy products in your diet, you should try to cut down and replace these staples with other ingredients.

THE DORCHESTER HOTEL (The Dorchester, 53 Park Lane, London W1A 2HJ, phone 020 7629 8888) is one of London's most famous hotels, having starred in countless films and media shoots and its reputation is second to none. "THE DORCH" is known not only for its beautiful suites (especially the one which starred in the Rom Com "WIMBLEDON" in 2004!) but for the high quality of the food served in its high profile restaurants and throughout the hotel. I always choose THE DORCHESTER's elegant ballroom for all my charity and political balls because I know that I can rely on the food being superb even when served to 450 people at once, thanks to their excellent banqueting manager, GARETH BUSH and executive chef HENRY BROSI and team. As executive chef of THE DORCHESTER, the talented HENRY is in charge of all the hotel's kitchens including THE GRILL ROOM, THE DORCHESTER BAR and THE KRUG ROOM (the beautifully designed private dining room) as well as the banqueting department and room service. The award winning MR BROSI has worked at many of the world's other top hotels including THE WALDORF ASTORIA in New York, THE SACHER in Vienna and CLARIDGE'S in London and is passionate about his work. He has prepared a superb three-course meal especially for us containing no wheat or dairy ingredients with an optional low-dairy-content "yoghurt sorbet" for those of us who are not on a strict "no wheat or dairy" diet and just want to cut down considerably.

Luckily nowadays there is an immense variety of gluten free products on the market. A large selection can be found at any of the branches of the wonderful chain of health food shops HOLLAND & BARRETT. For a special treat of hand-made organic foods, visit www.crayves.co.uk and find their list of stockists. They are wholesalers of the most delicious special range of gluten, soya, dairy, sugar and wheat free hand-made products freshly produced daily.

Kinesiology

Do we really all know what foods are good for us and what are not?

You may need to try kinesiology, an alternative therapy through which you can find out which foods agree or disagree with your individual body (or "temple" as you must now learn to call it!)

This is how JILL HOPLEY, kinesiologist at London's leading alternative medicine clinic, THE HALE CLINIC (7 Park Crescent, London, W1B 1PF, phone 020 7631 0156, web-

THREE COURSE NO WHEAT NO DAIRY MENU

by Executive Chef, The Dorchester, Mr Henry Brosi

Course one: Starter

Salad of English asparagus with summer leaves and truffle dressing   *Serves 10*

INGREDIENTS

40 pieces English asparagus spears
50 g fresh summer truffle
80 g salad plûche

DRESSING

100 ml extra virgin olive oil
10 ml Champagne vinegar
150 ml chicken sediment (roasting juice)
10 pieces edible flowers
100 g mixed herbs (cerfeuil, chives, flat leaf parsley, tarragon)
200 g micro sprouts (beetroot, pea shoots, onion shoots)

METHOD

1 Method for the truffle dressing:
Warm up the chicken sediment and reduce by one third.
Use half of the truffle and chop very finely. Add to the sediment.
Gently whisk the olive oil into the sediment mixture and then add the Champagne vinegar.
Cover with cling film and allow to infuse for about one hour before using.

2 Peel and blanch the asparagus and refresh in iced water. Re-heat the asparagus gently until nice and warm.

Strain and then toss in a little of the truffle dressing and season well.
Form little bouquets of the summer leaves, herbs and micro shoots and season with salt and pepper.
Arrange the asparagus spears in a diamond shape on the plate.

3 Arrange the salad mixture in the middle. Drizzle the dressing over the salad and around the plate.
Using a truffle slicer, slice the truffle over the salad and decorate each plate with an edible flower. Serve.

Course two: Main course

Steamed fillet of turbot "duglere" with balsamic reduction and yellow pepper sauce   *Serves 10*

INGREDIENTS

10 pieces turbot (160 g) (skinless)
1 kg plum tomatoes
300 g shallots
¼ litre olive oil
80 g garlic, peeled
1 sprig thyme
1 sprig rosemary
400 ml yellow pepper coulis
100 ml balsamic reduction
50 g basil
500 g spinach
60 g Jersey royal potatoes

METHOD

Season the turbot with salt and pepper.
Blanch tomatoes briefly to peel skins, then slice into wedges. Remove seeds.
Place tomatoes onto baking trays with olive oil, garlic, herbs. Season. Cook slowly in oven at 100°C.
Confit the peeled shallots.
Place tomatoes on top of fish, approximately six pieces per fish. Garnish with shallot on top.
Steam fish in oven for about 5–6 minutes.
Pipe balsamic reduction into a big square, very thinly.

Sauté the spinach and place on the middle of the plate.
Place fish in the middle and serve with pepper coulis and potatoes.

Yellow pepper coulis   *Makes 1 litre of coulis*

INGREDIENTS

1 kg yellow peppers
200 g shallots
1 clove garlic, crushed
2 tbsp extra virgin olive oil
250 ml vegetable stock
1 sprig thyme
salt, freshly ground pepper

METHOD

Roast the peppers in the oven until the skins blister slightly.
Put the peppers into ice water to peel off the skin.
Halve the peppers and deseed them. Then cut them into chunky pieces.
Sauté the chopped shallots in a sauté

pan without colouring and then add the peppers and garlic.
Add the vegetable stock.
Cook to a syrup consistency and infuse with the thyme.
Using a high speed blender, blend the pepper mix to a smooth consistency.
Check the seasoning.

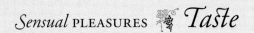
Course three: Dessert

Poached exotic fruits with passion fruit coulis and lychee yoghurt sorbet   *Serves 10*

EXOTIC FRUITS	PASSION FRUIT COULIS	LYCHEE YOGHURT SORBET *(20 portions)*
300 g pineapple	*100 g eggs*	*250 g lychee purée*
400 g mango	*90 g sugar*	*10 g mango juice*
400 g paw paw	*100 g passion fruit purée*	*50 g plain natural yoghurt*
1 litre orange juice	*10 g vanilla pod*	*5 g lemon juice*
1 stick lemon grass	Bring the purée and vanilla pod to the boil.	*50 g stock syrup*
Boil the orange juice and lemon grass and allow to infuse.	Whisk the eggs and sugar together and add to the purée. Bring back to the boil whisking continuously.	Make a purée using the fresh lychees. Add all the other ingredients and freeze in the ice-cream machine.
Cut the fruits into ½ cm cubes. Pour over the lukewarm juice and allow to soak overnight.	Cook out for a few minutes.	
Drain and pass into rings (1 cm high x 4 cm in diameter).	Cover with cling film and allow to cool.	

site www.haleclinic.com) describes this interesting technique: *"Using muscle testing, kinesiology addresses the four components of the human body – the mental/emotional realm, the dietary and chemical factors, structural considerations and life force energy – and corrects the imbalances, restoring well-being.*

Since my kinesiology sessions with the HALE CLINIC I have learned that too much wheat, dairy and sugar do not agree with moi personally and I have ditched my Super Tasty Golden Toasted Wheaty Flakes in favour of good old gluten free porridge oats and have replaced milk and sugar with soy milk and honey. I only had to cut out wheat, dairy and sugar for a month before gradually reintroducing them into my diet but in moderation: not such a   sacrifice really.

It is not that difficult to cut out wheat and dairy products whether you are eating out or at home. For instance at our HOT GOSSIP favourite, "FRANKIE'S Italian Bar and Grill", (3 Yeoman's Row, off Brompton Road, Knightsbridge, SW3 2AL, phone 020 7590 9999 – part of the world-wide group owned by champion jockey FRANKIE DETTORI and restaurateur and chef *par excellence* MARCO-PIERRE WHITE) I usually have "Parma Ham with Figs or Avocado", "Tuna alla Mediterraneo" and "Champagne-poached Strawberries" (are your mouths watering, ladies who lunch?)

I always seem to order this menu even when I am not watching my wheat and dairy intake simply because those dishes are delicious, nutritious and, as the charming MR WHITE says, "for skinny birds". If you have to give up sugar as well, even if just for a month, it is a harder task: you will just have to eat your strawberries raw. (Again not a big sacrifice with such a naturally delicious fruit.) Sadly giving up sugar means abandoning wine, so no champagne-poached anything for a little while and do not go mad when you return to a "normal" diet. The good news is that, while you are "off" sugar, you can drink vodka. I would never normally recommend drinking spirits of any kind but if you cannot drink wine and champagne for a month you will probably need a little alternative treat every now and then!

Some people have serious food allergies: shellfish or nuts, for example, can kill and even mushrooms can make an allergic person extremely ill. If you think you may be allergic to certain foods consult your doctor at once; he or she can refer you for allergy testing which will sort out the problem.

Once you have found out which foods are good for you (and your family if, like me, you are a housewife and mother and need to make sure that your loved ones' "temples" are as healthy as your own) then go for it. Learn to enjoy the sensual pleasure of eating delicious but nutritious food which will build you up and morph you into the fit, healthy and glowing goddess that you can be. If, like me, you veer towards vegetarian, good for you: the animals will thank you. There are lots of marvellous veggie dishes around nowadays with "vegetarian options" available at most restaurants and events. It is always easy to find vegetarian starters, (and desserts, of course!) but finding a main course which is as satisfying as meat for friends and family who may not be of the veggie persuasion is much harder. You will need to bulk up with eggs, cheese, pasta or rice.

Celebrity TV chef JEAN-CHRISTOPHE NOVELLI (NOVELLI AT AUBERGE DU LAC, Brocket Hall International Ltd., Welwyn, Herts. AL8 7XG, phone 01707 368 888; NOVELLI ACADEMY, Crouchmoor Farm, Stony Lane, Tea Green, Luton LU2 8PS, phone

01582 454 070; NOVELLI IN THE CITY, Capital Club, 14 Abchurch Lane, London EC4 7B, phone 020 7717 0088) is renowned for his delicious and unusual dishes. Opposite is the recipe for his yummy scrummy "Classic Pipérade" which is made with softly boiled eggs but, as JEAN-CHRISTOPHE told me, tastes just as delicious with either penne or risotto.

French heart throb NOVELLI is definitely into sensual pleasures and described to me how cooking can be a sensually pleasurable experience: listen up, would be kitchen goddesses. *"Cooking is like sex for me. I cook with all of my five senses. Apart from tasting, smelling and looking at the food, you have to feel your way. When you are looking at one thing cooking, listen for the changing sounds of other dishes as they bubble and hiss and sing to you. Above all listen to your instincts."*

Alternatives to diet

Nutrition is big business all over the world these days and rightly so. You simply cannot achieve total good health if you do not care what you put inside your "temple". Below and overleaf are excerpts of a report which will really make you think from PETER COX, nutritionist at London's renowned HB HEALTH (12 Beauchamp Place, Knightsbridge, SW3 1NZ, phone 020 7838 0765) which specialises in anti-ageing, a subject close to all our hearts.

NOVELLI'S CLASSIC PIPÉRADE   *Serves 4*

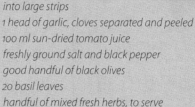

INGREDIENTS
4 warm soft-boiled eggs, halved
vegetables for the pipérade
100 ml olive oil
1 large courgette, sliced at an angle
1 medium aubergine, sliced at an
angle and then each slice halved
12 small shallots, peeled
8 baby fennel, trimmed
2 red peppers, deseeded and cut
into large strips
1 head of garlic, cloves separated and peeled
100 ml sun-dried tomato juice
freshly ground salt and black pepper
good handful of black olives
20 basil leaves
handful of mixed fresh herbs, to serve

METHOD
1 Prepare the Pipérade Vegetables: heat the olive oil in pan. Add the vegetables, garlic and sun-dried tomato juice and season. Cover with a tight-fitting lid and leave on low heat until the vegetables are just soft to the touch.
2 Remove the vegetables from the heat and add the olives and basil to warm through.
3 Carefully arrange the vegetables on four plates with the soft-boiled eggs and serve garnished with fresh herbs.

EATING "UP" THE EVOLUTIONARY SCALE
from Peter Cox

A woman's role?
Like it or not women have assumed responsibility for a family's eating habits. Whether you are mother, wife or daughter or all of these, you probably have more influence over your family's eating patterns than your male counterparts.

For the first time in western history we are witnessing a decline in collective health. For many of us there is a good chance we will die at ages younger than our parents and an increasing chance our children will die before us. This is not about years alive though, it's about the life in our years. Have we really abandoned vitality for time at the computer, workstation or play station?

Our nutritional health is stratified not by economic or even genetic success but by

choice. Think about it. Where do you want you and your family to be on the nutritional evolutionary scale? You have the opportunity to drag yourself and your family from your current health plateaux to at least the next rung of the nutritional evolutionary ladder.

Cack gobblers and gutter snackers
Cack gobblers and gutter snackers inhabit street corners, attracted to the fast food outlets. In our supermarkets their trolleys are full of plastic. Their food shopping converging with cosmetics and detergents, they had just as well suck on deodorant and swill washing liquid for the goodness they can derive from their shiny processed foods. What they eat is not food, was never food and has no nutritional value. These

people are held together by structural anti-nutrients and disease.
Fruit and vegetable count – SFA!
Quality protein count – are you kidding?
Water count – is that what we use to wash the car?

Toxin slaves
Toxin slaves are slaves not to other men but to their masters, the commercial dictators who control their slaves through toxic foods and drugs. The slaves' dependencies are exploited for all it is worth in order to feed the money making machinery of western industry.

Now refined sugars and hydrogenated fats, the toxic corollaries of real foods are fed to the slaves to feed their innate cravings for essential nutrition. Starved of their vital nourishment the Toxin Slaves uncontrollably crave these nearly foods until they become bloated and fetid, cantankerous and bilious until they receive their next fix.

They inhabit supermarkets, pharmacies and doctors' surgeries, so regular at their GPs that they block book appointments and possess open prescriptions. Their trolleys and baskets filled with brightly packaged products with promises of huge pleasure and eternal health. Do not worry about how sick you become, there is always a food to make you feel better and a drug to cure you. So conned, so sad.

Fruit and veg count – one per day
Quality protein count – one per day
Water count – only as soda.

Institutionalised eaters

They think because they are paying "top dollar" for their restaurant meal that they are being well nourished. Few have the courage to question the quality of their food. Built around cheap carbohydrates this food is adulterated to a point of debase, caked in a slime of reconstituted sauce yet garnished with a little broccoli or a few green beans or a countable number of peas or a stiff piece of lettuce and a slice of tomato. "Five portions of fruit and vegetables", the World Health Organization cry, yet our Institutionalised Eaters brag about the consumption of that wilted old piece of lettuce.

The Institutionalised Eaters are recognisable by definition. They inhabit not only our schools, old people's homes and hospitals, they also occupy the city coffee shops and sandwich bars, sit in nouveau cuisine restaurants staring hungrily at the gutter snacker's glowing potato snacks and the battlefields of industry and war. Identifiable by their hope and progressive malnutrition.

Fruit and veg count – one to two per day
(but not necessarily identifiable as such).
Quality protein count – one per day.
Water count – mainly as tea.

Informed consumers

The Informed Consumers have read the newspaper articles, have absorbed the government recommendations, read the most important popular texts and some have even heard of Patrick Holford. They have negotiated the Internet and visit their GPs informed and able to argue their case. They are also intelligent enough to know when to listen to their doctors and when not. They have recognised the benefits of healthy eating and have incorporated it into their balanced lives.

They eat five portions of fruit and vegetables per day because that constitutes the balanced meals they have been consuming since the Roman or Norman invasions. They are well nourished and understand the benefits but most importantly this is what they do because it has always worked and there is no reason to change. They often eat organically, not because they understand and value the benefits but because they can afford it.

Informed Consumers might use supplements but tend towards conservatism. They might take something, especially if it is a traditional remedy or they have read about its efficacy for a member of the royal family or an admired celebrity. Important to this group though is that the supplement must not replace the food and traditional well grown, prepared and cooked foods.

You will find this group in garden centres, picking out the seeds to grow their own. They curmudgeonly glide around Waitrose and Selfridges' food halls downloading the details of organic produce into those supposedly time saving gadgets which bleep a knowing bleep. Notice them at bookshops thumbing the cookbooks along with the travel guides – just stocking up on some exotic nutrition.

Fruit and veg count – four to five per day.
Quality protein count – two per day.
Water count – one litre per day.

Space age eaters

So to the top of the evolutionary nutrition tree. Space Age Eaters can come from any social or economic group. They recognise the concept of bio individuality and have identified their own strengths and weaknesses. This has been done through testing and/or with behavioural experimentation. Food is messaging and the Space Age Eaters have their "receivers switched on". They know which foods work for them and which don't. What is more they can manipulate their nutrition according to their changing environments and requirements. This method of nourishment identifies with ancient practices, including ayurverdic, oriental and naturopathic, all of which utilise food as primary medicine.

It is not by chance that this group appear younger, fitter, healthier and more effective than their counterparts it is the culmination of their objective and determined efforts, either innate or structured to make the most of what they have. Space Age Eaters, if not examining the increasing evidence available about the benefits of specific diets and nutrients in relation to specific requirements, seek guidance from the new wave of informed practitioners often working in integrated health practices. These practitioners are not constrained by a single discipline but incorporate, as far as is possible, all that is best from all forms of healthcare, ancient and modern.

Space Age Eaters are recognisable at the offices of nutritionists and other practitioners but also via their use of the Net. They read widely, listen intently and most importantly apply what they know carefully, detecting the signals their bodies produce in order to fine-tune their nutrition and their internal environments. The only down side is due to being exceptional, although their peculiarity is tempered by their vitality and mental performance. It is not about being the best, it is about being as good as you can be.

Fruit and veg count – six to ten per day.
Quality protein count – three per day.
Water count – two to three litres per day.

Summary

Having identified where you and your family sit on the evolutionary nutrition scale, what is most important to understand is that you can drag you and your family up the scale. We have fairly equal access to plenty of good quality foods. Our supermarkets are awash with not only dietary cack but also nutritious foods.

Eating well is no longer enough. We can all eat and indeed nourish ourselves optimally. Using the fruit and veg, quality protein and water counts you can work your way up the scale. A step or two will make a "world of difference" to how you feel. You can all become Space Age Eaters.

As a helpful guide to those of you attempting to improve your nutrition but struggling with commercial and government misinformation, here are a few handy hints:

Processed foods – place firmly in the bin anything with more than three ingredients.

Low fat foods – avoid like the plague, they have had their nutrition removed.

Low sugar foods – avoid like the plague.

Bread – only if you like breaking wind!

Fish – eat because it is brain food.

Red meat – eat as much as you would expect to catch as a hunter.

Water – drink until you are no longer thirsty.

Full fat foods – eat because they contain essential nutriments.

Yoghurt drinks – switch to natural yoghurt and vegetables.

Fruit – eat what is fresh and in season.

Vegetables – eat what is fresh and in season or grow your own.

Vegetarianism – bloody hard work.

Alcohol – drink it as far as you can handle it.

Cakes and biscuits – grow up.

Chocolate – only the proper stuff.

Supplements – buy the best you can afford but only the ones you need.

Sweets, soft drinks and refined snacks – have you not read this report yet?

So now we know! Food combining is another important consideration for both health and losing weight. Below are PETER COX's thoughts.

I also asked PETER whether he thought boiling or microwaving were better for heating both food and water (we are coming to the benefits of hot water in the next chapter). This is what he said:

"On the balance of evidence microwaving is probably best for food and perhaps water. Boiling destroys key nutrients and dumps minerals from water. The jury is still out on microwaving; it appears to kill enzymes but then so does all cooking."

Personally I always try to steam my vegetables and recommend buying a steamer and keeping it short and sweet to retain all the goodness. Stir frying quickly is also very healthy if you do not overdo the oil.

FOOD COMBINING
from Peter Cox

The concept of food combining, better described as the de-combining of foods was originally developed by Dr William Hay during the early years of the last century. He developed his ideas primarily as a treatment of his own malaise and after succeeding in treating his own considerable health problems extended his dietary treatments to his own patients.

Hay's original work suggested people's health problems emanated from the accumulation of toxins produced by poor digestion. He attributed excess toxicity to the over consumption of meat, the over consumption of refined carbohydrates, disregard of the rules of digestion and the effects of constipation. Hay's original work showed that improved digestion was associated with better health. As a by-product of his recommendations people also lost weight. Hay's ideas were modernised in Doris Grant's 1984 book *Food Combining for Health*. Since then food combining has become synonymous with weight loss but

remains a concept more geared towards establishing a fundamental change in digestive function, and with that, health.

The rules of food combining are very simple and describe a return to a "more natural" way of eating. This involves:

■ Not mixing starches and sugars with protein rich foods at the same meal.

■ Eating protein rich, fat rich and carbohydrate rich foods in modest quantities.

■ Ensuring vegetables, including salads and fruit make up the bulk of the diet.

■ The avoidance of refined sugars, primarily white sugar and white flour.

■ Avoidance of over-eating.

It is difficult to argue against the logic of Hay's recommendations and most people are likely to benefit to some extent by incorporating some, if not all, of his suggestions into their diets. In a "nutshell" over-loading of our guts tends to occur when we eat sugar rich foods (bread, sugar, pasta, rice, cereals and potatoes) with protein rich foods, especially flesh foods

(meat, fish, dairy produce and eggs). This overwhelming of our guts leads to incomplete digestion and the development of toxic by-products. These toxins have an adverse effect on the body which can lead to inflammation and disease.

Whilst this isn't "Rocket Science", most traditional meals have developed to combine proteins with complex carbohydrates, such as meat and potatoes in the UK, bread and beans in South America, meat with rice in China, pulses and rice in the Indian sub-continent and pasta with meat/fish in Mediterranean regions. Digestive problems are most likely to have developed with "convenient" eating. The fewer meals we eat the more we want to pack our major sources of protein and starch into one meal, with consequent digestive impairment. The more concentrated the sources of starch/sugar and protein/fat the greater the demands on our powers of digestion. Our digestive systems clearly work better when they are not over-taxed.

Taste

2
DRINK

Wε all know that we should drink two litres of water a day to achieve perfect health. This feels like hard work sometimes, especially in winter when one is not so naturally thirsty but do drink as much as you can: one litre is better than none. The debate about bottled water versus tap water rumbles on. I tend to drink bottled spa water if I can in London where the water is rumoured to have been circulated through the system seven times but tap water if I happen to be in the mountains or in a spa area.

Water, soft drinks and juice

As it is not always easy or appetising to consume two litres of cold water in the winter months, try drinking hot boiled or microwaved water instead. Warm, body temperature water is actually better for your digestion and drinking it warm will make you feel as if you are having a hot drink, which you are and is much better for you than the ubiquitous coffee and tea, which are bad for the jolly old cellulite. If you are really posh, as JOANNA LUMLEY would say, you can pop a slice of lemon in which is very cleansing and makes you feel as if you are at an exclusive health farm: GRAYSHOTT, FOREST MERE or CHAMPNEYS maybe? Some unscrupulous cafe owners add a twist of lemon rind, call it a "canareno" and charge you £4.00 for it; this is something I always say *is* safe to try at home!

In the summer it is much easier to drink two litres of water daily and once you have consumed your quota, you can treat yourself to a delicious fruit, ginger, camomile or mint tea, all of which are much better than coffee or normal tea for the digestion, the nerves and the cellulite. Water is cleansing and de-toxing for the body and is best drunk between meals to avoid bloating; if you are dieting a large glass of water will help to fill you up with absolutely no calorific value whatsoever, unlike most things which pass our lips! It is actually supposed to be better not to drink anything at all with food but this is anti-social and inconvenient.

The only problem with drinking a lot of water is that you will need to have several "pit stops" to get rid of it. This is the general idea: you are flushing out all the toxins from your body including naughty foods and alcohol. However it is inconvenient and will remind the mothers amongst us of pregnancy. Never mind, drinking water and getting rid of it is good for you. Just do not drink too much of your daily quota in the afternoon and evening if you want an uninterrupted night's sleep; in fact I usually drink my last glass (of eight if possible) of water before six p.m. Having drunk your quota you will feel virtuous and that is when you can treat yourself to something altogether more sensually pleasurable.

Many dieters rely on carbonated drinks to fill them up or as an alcohol substitute but although "sodas" are delicious and often have no calories at all, they are seriously bad for skin, teeth and cellulite. These drinks are a crutch you should really ditch if you want to achieve perfect health; if you are really hooked, please go the moderation route.

Fruit juice in cartons is much better than sodas but, if you want to be really healthy and get rid of any cellulite, you should get a power juicer and juice your own fresh fruit and vegetables: carrots, celery and beetroot all make delicious fresh drinks but forget tomatoes, they are just not juicing material. Fruit juices are also not good for the teeth when drunk in between meals, as they contain too much natural sugar and it is always advisable to brush your teeth after consuming anything sweet if you can.

Dental advice

After all it is impossible to look like a health goddess without a set of sparkling white, hopefully natural, teeth; if you have really abused your teeth over the years and have, God forbid, been a smoker (we are coming to that subject soon) you may need to get your teeth bleached.

LOOKING AFTER YOUR TEETH

from Mr Malcolm Freiberger

Looking after your dental health is important because you don't want gum and tooth disease but you do want a healthy and attractive smile. You have an important role as a co-therapist with your dentist and the following advice will help you.

Please minimise the intake of sugary foods and drinks, and dietary acids. Limit their consumption to meal times, avoiding them between meals to reduce the risks of decay and erosion. Dietary acids are found in fruit, fruit juice, yoghurt, carbonated water, carbonated soft drinks, wine, vinegar, and effervescent vitamin C tablets. Avoid biting on boiled sweets or other very hard food which could fracture your teeth and their restorations.

I routinely advise patients with crowns or veneers on their front teeth to be careful when eating bread rolls, corn-on-the-cob, spare ribs, raw fruit and vegetables as these types of foods are more likely to cause the porcelain to fracture. This can easily be avoided by cutting up these foods before chewing them.

Home care removes bacterial plaque and minimises the chances of decay and gum disease. Gum disease is a bacterial infection due to the accumulation of bacterial plaque on the surfaces of our teeth. The plaque bacteria provoke an inflammatory response called gingivitis which is typified by gum bleeding. Gingivitis is a reversible, curable disease which will disappear if the bacterial film is removed by effective oral hygiene at home supported by maintenance in the surgery.

Gingivitis is a common condition and is reversible but about 10 to 20% of us are susceptible to the plaque and develop periodontitis which involves gum damage and the loss of bone around the roots of some of our teeth which makes them become loose. We do not yet know why gingivitis progresses to periodontitis, a change which will be detected by your dentist who will then be able to initiate treatment to control the disease.

I recommend brushing your teeth for two minutes twice a day with fluoride toothpaste, and using floss and interdental brushes once a day to help keep your teeth clean and your gums healthy.

Cigarette smoking is very harmful because it makes us more susceptible to gum disease and serious diseases such as mouth cancer, particularly in combination with alcohol.

I think prevention is better than expensive time-consuming treatment and recommend that you and your dentist should meet at agreed intervals for recall and maintenance appointments to screen for oral disease and maintain the health of your gums and teeth.

Above is a report from MR MALCOLM FREIBERGER, BDS LDSRCS MFGDP, (9a Portland Place, London, W1, phone 020 7636 8495) one of the West End's most respected dental practitioners who also practises cosmetic dentistry.

If you have not, in fact, looked after your teeth or you are more mature, they may become rotten and you may have to have them removed (yes, really! This is deadly serious). Dentures are the obvious answer but not an attractive option at any age: save up your dosh and plump for implants instead. MR FREIBERGER has implanted several patients with total success and two of my mates (who are *not* old, I stress) who now have implants look great.

DR SHIRAZ GULAMALI, BDS, LDSRCS, MSC, FDSRCPS has a practice exclusive to Periodontics and Dental Implants (12 Upper Wimpole Street, London, W1G 6LW, phone 020 7486 2466 or 020 7935 9511, www.gumsandimplants.co.uk). He is a registered Specialist in Periodontics, with an extensive background in oral surgery and restorative dentistry. He qualified from Guys Dental Hospital in 1980 and entered private referral practice in 1988 having completed various postgraduate qualifications.

Dr Gulamali lectures in the UK and abroad. He told me:

TOOTH LOSS
from Dr Shiraz Gulamali

The consequences of tooth loss, usually through dental decay, failing restorations or periodontal (gum) disease can be dramatic, both psychologically as well as physically. Patients who suffer tooth loss, whether single or multiple units, become acutely aware of their functional compromise and accompanying cosmetic embarrassment.

Not only does tooth loss result in premature ageing as facial contours are affected, it also brings into focus one's oral health which, in turn, is a major factor associated with good general health.

One may want to consider dental implants to replace failing or missing teeth. The process of replacing missing teeth with implants deals with both the functional aspects, as well as the aesthetic demands of each individual case. The reconstruction of a natural smile is a form of art, highly dependent on the clinician's multidisciplinary training, professional development and personal skills.

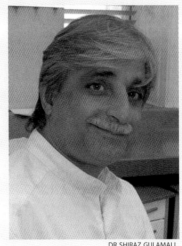

DR SHIRAZ GULAMALI

Today, individuals in modern society are more than ever geared toward high expectations of good health and are living longer lives. Our concern with facial profiles are very much part of our changing attitudes. Favourable facial contours are created by the unique relationship between the lips,

gums and teeth. All are constituent parts of a harmonious smile. Both teeth and implants have a crucial role to play in maintaining natural facial contours. The chronic full denture-wearer is an unfortunate example of someone who has suffered the collapse of the lower half of the face. Dental implants, together with other procedures offered by disciplines such as periodontal plastic surgery, can offset such collapses. They offer the individual the opportunity to have replacement teeth that currently perform as close to natural teeth as possible. They affect not only significant cosmetic improvements, but also allow better enjoyment of food, easier digestion and less troublesome speech. Above all, implants maintain facial profile. With this comes the tremendous psychological advantage of being able to live life with confidence.

It is always gratifying to see a patient leave the practice with a mouth that is not only functional, but also aesthetically pleasing.

Alcoholic drinks

Then of course there is "the demon drink": alcohol. There is no more sensual taste pleasure to me than the bubbles of a vintage champagne on my tongue; or indeed a chilled, dry white wine. For some people it is a full bodied, fruity red wine, for others a smoky malt whisky or a sweet liqueur. There is nothing quite like alcohol as a mood elevator. Drugs and pills are simply out of the question if you want to be a health goddess but alcohol in moderation is acceptable and eminently sociable.

Apparently some hospitals and homes are now advocating a glass of red wine a day for the elderly as being "good for the haemoglobin". HOT GOSSIP UK'S consultant GP, DR RICHARD HART (020 8952 5536) confirms: *"Red wine contains an antioxidant which reduces cholesterol so it is, indeed, good for you on one level at least"*. Well, surprise, surprise. Or as DAVID WEST, entrepreneur, TV producer, proprietor of HEY JO nightclub (91 Jermyn Street, St James's, W1, phone 020 7930 3222) and the UK's biggest

wine importer (EASTENDERS' PRIME WINES, phone 020 7930 52372) would say "I told you so!"

Too much alcohol is, however, bad for your digestion, your skin and the whites of your eyes so do be moderate in your drinking. Two glasses a day of your favourite tipple is plenty and will keep you sparkling without making you comatose! We can all "tie one on" sometimes but if you begin to drink seriously and become addicted to alcohol (all too easily done) you should seek professional help super-pronto.

DR ANDREW STRIGNER, MB, BS, MFHom, Fellow of the Royal Society of Medicine, Fellow of the Medical Society of London, Vice President of the McCarrison Society (for the study of the relationship of Health and Nutrition), Member of the Institute of the Study of Delinquency, author of *Healthy Eating and Common Sense – Food is mostly harmless* (phone: 020 7935 4543), told me about alcohol dependency and addiction. See panel on the next page.

Alcohol and hypnotherapy

Hypnotherapist VALERIE AUSTIN specialises in the treatment of alcohol addiction with her Asocial Alcohol Program. VALERIE says hundreds of people have sought her help for alcohol addiction and you should not be embarrassed about it. If you are shy, however, try Valerie's self hypnosis technique described in chapter one.

For those of you who live in or near the Totteridge area of London, DEBORAH D'ARCY (07939 479 420) is a healer who has had an extraordinarily high success rate hypnotising both alcohol and smoking addicts. Like most proper healers, DEBORAH does not charge for her healing and is also a gifted psychic and medium. Many people, especially devout Christians, do not approve of this sort of thing but I would be derelict in my duty if I did not mention psychics as they are so popular nowadays and can actually bring both comfort and fun to people's lives. You must go to a good one, of course, who really has the gift of clairvoyance and is not just a charlatan.

Two of the best and most respected (and my favourite) psychics in London are VALENTIN BORISSOV (118 Piccadilly, London, W1, phone 020 7569 6815) and PETER LEE (10 Linden Gardens, Notting Hill, W2, phone 020 7221 1238).

But I digress: back to the demon drink. If you would feel deprived and antisocial by not drinking at all, then go the moderation route. As with so many things in life, moderation is the key to imbibing. You do not have to be completely teetotal to remain healthy and beautiful: a couple of glasses of wine or champagne a day will not hurt you if you are not an addict and, as we heard from DR RICHARD HART in the previous chapter, red wine is actually quite good for you. I myself underwent hypnotherapy with VALERIE AUSTIN to bring my drinking down to just two glasses a day or at any one time and it worked perfectly for me. Two glasses with food is manageable; I can still drive and look after children safely but I feel more lively and sociable than if I were absolutely teetotal.

ALCOHOL DEPENDENCY/ADDICTION

from Dr Andrew Strigner

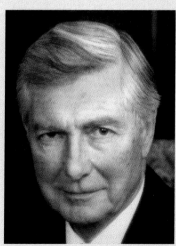

DR ANDREW STRIGNER

Alcohol seems to have appeared in all cultures in some form for thousands of years: presumably, at first accidentally, by consumption of naturally fermenting over-ripe fruit; later by deliberate production.

In pharmacological terms, alcohol is a cellular depressant – reducing mental and physical skills. Because it also acts as a dis-inhibitor, it can reduce tension and induce a sense of calm, but in a person of angry disposition can lead to violent behaviour.

As a result, there are today cultural differences. Some societies accept its "moderate use" as a social aid (this requires careful education "within the family" from early childhood). Others, on philosophical or religious grounds, impose a total ban.

Chronic over indulgence in alcohol can in some susceptible individuals lead to addiction and always liver and/or brain damage, with severe incapacity – and death.

Some cases of addiction may relate to the constituents of the drink and not to the alcohol i.e. an individual who is grain intolerant may become addicted to beer or whisky, but not to wine. Removal of grains from the diet improves that individual's sense of well-being with the loss of the addiction.

Where alcohol is a problem to the individual, whether physical or mental, there is no alternative but to stop its use entirely.

Taste

3

SMOKING, DRUGS,
MEDICATION, VITAMINS, ET AL.

SMOKING is not just a taste, it is an addiction. There is no way you can be completely healthy if you smoke, it is simply the worst. Apart from the obvious risk of lung cancer, smoking ages the skin and causes nasty little lines above the lips. Furthermore it is not exactly sensual for your breath, hair, clothes and home to smell like an old ashtray. The gorgeous MARLENE DIETRICH may have looked and sounded like a goddess with her sexy cigarette holder and gravelly voice but, if you try it, you may not be the sweetest smelling star in the firmament. We will address this problem further in our "smell" section but, for the moment, can I just advise you to stop smoking now? Yesterday, in fact. Remember that your cigarettes can also kill innocent non-smokers through passive smoking.

Giving up smoking was one of the hardest things I have ever done, but one of the most worthwhile. If, like me, you do not have much will power and the patches and gum have not worked, you may need hypnotherapy. As with alcohol addiction, if you cannot get to our hypnotherapist VALERIE AUSTIN or one of her staff or colleagues for treatment, you can try her self hypnosis method mentioned in chapter one and "suggest" yourself out of smoking.

I do not have to tell you that all hard drugs are terrible for your health and your looks so if you are addicted you must seek professional help and I suggest that you actually check in to a clinic and stay there until you are completely cured; this is sometimes also necessary for severe cases of alcohol addiction. The best-known rehab centre in the UK is probably THE PRIORY in Roehampton, London (020 8876 8261) where the rich, the famous and the seriously addicted go to dry out but there are now centres all over the country and your GP can refer you.

Soft drugs and too much medication should also be avoided; marijuana and Valium can both atrophy your brain if taken over a long period of time. Most sleeping pills and painkillers can be addictive, so try to take herbal remedies where possible. Insomnia can affect you at any time in your life, especially if you are stressed or going through hormonal changes. Hot milk or Horlicks does not always crack it and counting sheep will drive you to distraction! Insomnia is another problem which can be cured by hypnotherapy, as mine was by VALERIE AUSTIN.

Even the healthiest people can succumb to the common cold or cough and Day Nurse, Night Nurse and Benilyn all do the business but can make you very irritable if taken for long periods. Antibiotics should only be taken in extreme cases as they lose their efficacy if taken regularly for the tiniest little sniffle. Personally I do take a flu shot from my GP, DR MCKEOWN (7 Kynance Place, London, SW7, phone 020 7581 3040 if you happen to be doctor-less in Kensington) every autumn but, if you have never had flu, you may not need any preventative treatment.

Nowadays everyone is very big on food supplements and many of them are great but if you eat well you should not really need to take too many vitamins and minerals. If you cannot always have a balanced diet, a daily multi-vitamin is advisable and taking large doses of Vitamin C definitely helps get over colds and flu. The best pill I have ever found for PMT is Oil of Evening Primrose and regular Calcium tablets will improve the state of your hair and nails. All these supplements can be found at your local supermarket, pharmacy or health food shop. While you are in the health food shop have a look around; there are all sorts of natural "alternative" remedies which really work. For instance if you suffer from arthritis or need an anti-inflammatory cure for any reason try BROMELAIN which is made from pineapples and will not upset the lining of your stomach like the "proper" medication. Or try XANGO, the delicious new "wonder" drink which is a natural anti-inflammatory made from the exotic mangosteen fruit (available from: 01329 280727 or: brianonline@tiscali.co.uk)

Some more of my personal favourites are:

- ❧ Arnica for bruises and to heal scars from the inside,
- ❧ Thuja for warts and veruccas, which are affecting more and more people at the moment and
- ❧ Ginger as an anti-inflammatory and for the digestion (ginger tea is especially soothing to the stomach after a large meal).

These are just a few magic remedies but the sheer amount of capsules and tablets on the shelves can be confusing and some pills need to be taken in a certain way. For instance tissue salts such as arnica, thuja, etc. should not be touched by hand: put them straight into your mouth from the bottle and let them dissolve on the tongue. Also it is important to be aware that 6c, for instance, is five times stronger than 30c as these salts are measured by dilution, not by strength.

You should always take advice from your GP or a good pharmacist before taking pills or applying potions willy nilly. I always check with my own doctor, DR MCKEOWN or HOT GOSSIP's consultant DR RICHARD HART before trying any new food supplement or homeopathic remedy either for myself or for my family. Plus I could not survive without my knowledgeable and diligent local pharmacist MAC PATEL (Parmay Pharmacy, 160 North End Road, West Kensington, W14 9PR, phone 020 7381 4376).

By the way if you are up in the Harley Street area for medical or beauty treatments, the most knowledgeable and diligent pharmacist in that area is MAHESH SONEJI (Madesil Pharmacy, 20 Marylebone High Street, London, W1U 4PB, phone 020 7935 3078).

Taste

4

EAT YOURSELF HEALTHY
DISEASE PREVENTION PLUS ANTI-AGEING,
MENOPAUSE & HORMONES

I F there is a history of cancer or heart disease in your family you need to look after yourself. Eating five portions of fresh fruit or veg daily is really important and please do not smoke or overdo the alcohol. If you have a problem remembering what foods you should eat and how much and/or want to encourage your family to "eat right", order a Rainbow Food Activity Chart from LEMONBURST (01273 558112) immediately. All the foods illustrated are listed on TV nutritionist DR GILLIAN MCKEITH's *Food Abundance* list and kids will have great fun using the cute re-useable stickers. Then I suggest you dust off the power juicer and the blender and treat yourself to lots of scrummy fresh juices and smoothies: definitely a sensual pleasure!

DR ANDREW STRIGNER is Vice President of the McCarrison Society (for the study of the relationship of Health and Nutrition). He gave me the following information which should inspire us all to bring down our cholesterol levels and protect ourselves from cancer and heart disease:

Cholesterol
"Cholesterol is vital to life – every cell in the body needs it to function – 70–80% being made in the body.

Raised cholesterol levels appear to be a 'western' disease, afflicting those societies that have adopted the style of eating prevailing in Britain and the US. High cholesterol is certainly a principal factor in coronary heart disease.

Ethnic societies, such as bushmen in the Kalahari desert and Australian aborigines living in their traditional style untouched by civilisation, all have low cholesterol levels and no problems with raised blood pressure, coronary heart disease or cancer. Their diet consists of a wide variety of wild vegetables, berries, fish and/or game meat and occasional eggs.

Similarly the Inuit (Eskimo) people, although denied access to vegetables for the greater part of the year, have similarly low cholesterol levels and no problems with high blood pressure, coronary, heart disease or cancer. Their diet consists of a very high proportion of marine foods – fish and animal – which contribute essential fatty acids which are also found in the diets of the bushmen and aboriginals but which are sorely lacking and out of balance in foods of so-called developed countries.

Levels of cholesterol are most quickly raised by intake of sugar, starches and excess of saturated fat – substances that were absent in the ancestral diet, but have appeared in increasing amounts since the advent of agriculture.

Regular, moderate physical exercise tends to lower raised cholesterol.

Regarding cancer, evidence from the International Cancer Research Foundation indicates that by eating correctly i.e. approaching that of our early ancestors, you reduce the risk of developing cancer by 40%. If you do not smoke and eat correctly, the risk is cut by 70%.

Other factors:

- *Environmental, e.g. diesel fumes from motor vehicles, chemicals used in industry (and nowadays in homes), magnetic radiation from nearby high voltage power lines, alpha and gamma radiation from radon gas trapped in houses lacking in ventilation or locations of granite soils as in the English West Country and medical X-rays.*

- *Genetic: probably the lowest."*

Stress can exacerbate disease, including heart disease and some types of cancer so keep away from stressful people and situations: this is my personal New Year's resolution every year!

We used to think that men were much more prone to heart disease but in today's world many more women seem to be suffering. Below is an interesting report from eminent Harley Street cardiovascular surgeon MR RAKESH UPPAL, BSc, MBCHB,

FRCS, (C/Th) (149 Harley Street, London, W1G 6DE, phone 020 7935 6397, www.thelondonclinic.co.uk, r.uppal@thelondonclinic.co.uk).

I recommend that you read *Stop Inflammation Now!* by cardiologist DR RICHARD FLEMING, ISBN 1583332006 published by Penguin about the twelve main causes of heart attack and stroke which includes his breakthrough plan to restore heart health: why simple diet and lifestyle changes can help prevent, treat and even reverse heart disease.

CORONARY HEART DISEASE

from Mr Rakesh Uppal

Coronary heart disease is becoming more common in women. The reasons are complex, but women are living longer and obesity and lack of exercise are more prevalent, resulting in a higher prevalence of diabetes. Worryingly in young women and teenagers the rates of smoking is actually rising. Women become especially susceptible to heart disease after the menopause, and the likelihood of dying from heart disease after the menopause is almost equal to that in men.

How do you recognise a heart attack? It is a common misconception that heart attacks are very painful. Typically heavy or tight chest discomfort develops over the centre of the chest and this may radiate to the arm, neck and jaw. In many patients there may be breathlessness, sweating or nausea.

Unfortunately in over 40% the presentation is not typical, and almost a third fail to recognise these symptoms thinking they are simply having "bad indigestion", resulting in a delay in presentation which can be very dangerous. In diabetics the situation is worse and up to a quarter of heart attacks may be truly silent.

With a heart attack the speed of hospitalisation is the key to a good outcome. 40% of patients with a heart attack die in the first hour of onset of symptoms, and the outlook of those arriving at hospital alive nowadays is good. If you think you might be developing heart symptoms then call for an emergency ambulance and avoid looking for your GP, phoning the NHS direct, or even driving yourself up to a hospital. The nearest hospital is always the best!

In most heart attacks a clot in the coronary artery is blocking the blood supply. Breaking down this clot and preventing a further clot is life saving and can limit the degree of damage to the heart's pumping efficiency. 300 mg of aspirin is the first drug administered followed usually by a "clot-busting" drug, though nowadays immediate balloon treatment and stenting are increasingly being considered when feasible.

Modern treatment after a heart attack involves a combination of three to four drugs, a change in lifestyle and an assessment of the risk of further heart attacks. Increasingly patients are being assessed earlier for further treatment with coronary stenting and bypass surgery. A cardiac ultrasound (echocardiogram) is used to assess the heart's pumping action and presence of leakage of the heart valves, and an angiogram is undertaken to assess the degree of narrowing of the coronary arteries. With one or two arteries narrowed, stenting tends to be favoured; however with more extensive or complex disease, particularly in diabetics, bypass surgery may be preferable. With significant valve leakage, repair or replacement of the valve surgically is usually the only option. Although bypass surgery is a major undertaking the risks nowadays are extremely low, of the order of 1–2%.

If the heart muscle has been badly damaged, then recovery is slower, and you should limit exercise and avoid sex and playing very strenuous sport for six weeks or until your cardiologist or rehabilitation co-ordinator is satisfied with your progress. After stabilisation

and surgery or stenting the more physically active you are the better, even for patients with severe heart muscle damage. Avoid smoking at all costs, and piling on the weight.

So how do you avoid this in the first place? Well we can't choose our parents, or stop the ageing process. You can however help yourself by not smoking at all – even one cigarette daily increases the risk of a heart attack by 40%, and 20 daily by 400%!! It is never too late to stop, and within a year of stopping the risk of a heart attack is reduced substantially.

Eat sensibly – reduce saturated fats, red or fatty meats and dairy products. Increase dietary mono and polyunsaturated fats instead. Increase fish intake, particularly oily types (salmon, mackerel, herring), and fresh vegetables – five portions or more really does help reduce risk of coronary heart disease, and also some cancers. Keep your weight down, as obesity is now recognised as an important risk factor in its own right.

Exercise three to four times weekly. A half hour session of brisk walking every other day, enough to cause a warm glow over the face and sweating is enough. Leaving the car behind, parking furthest away, involving the family in the exercise habit or finding a partner to exercise with all help in increasing physical activity and this will help shed a few pounds too over the years!

Alcohol is protective to the heart in moderation, but be careful as women are more prone to liver damage above 14 units per week.

Mental stress has also been recently shown to be an important risk factor for coronary heart disease. Look for ways to minimise stress to yourself, and those around you. Catching the next train, letting someone go past, being nice to your colleagues and having a positive outlook will do wonders not only for your heart but also for those around you.

The risks go up particularly after the menopause, and the current perspective is that HRT is probably more harmful than beneficial in this regard. Consider having cardiovascular screening after the age of 55, or after 45 if you have a strong family history of coronary heart disease and stroke or if you are diabetic. If you are diabetic, have a raised blood pressure or high cholesterol, then the risk of having a heart attack or stroke will inevitably be higher.

The lifestyle measures outlined become even more important, and coupled with appropriate drug treatment can postpone or prevent a cardiac event in a large majority of women.

If this is a tall order and you can't achieve all of this, then some success is definitely better than none!

Sometimes you may need to look further afield than your own country to find the right treatment for your particular condition. Dynamic entrepreneur DAVID WEST leads a very busy life as a TV producer, club owner and wine importer not to mention the fact that he has a hectic social life with a string of beautiful girlfriends to entertain! Something had to give and in this case it was DAVID's heart. Here he tells his story:

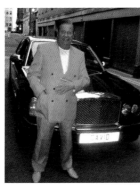

DAVID WEST

"Just before coming to Russia, I went for a blood check up in London and the English doctors said everything was fine. I had my routine check in Spain and they told me that my body and organisms were functioning properly – 100%. But the doctors in Russia came up with a different result. They didn't only scan my heart and take some blood tests but their check up system took 4–5 hours. It was very detailed and in-depth. They scanned every single corner of my body; the description of how my system was functioning took about 25 A4 pages – a mini-book! In that book they told me that I had had the disease for many years.

And another important thing – they are giving me pharmaceutical and natural products together. The English doctors never do that. I think that the Russian doctors probably are the best in the world! And the cost of this treatment which covers 21 days is less then the price that you'd pay for one day in the UK. And furthermore foreigners are treated the same as the Russians: we don't pay more because we have more!

It is too early to comment on my treatment because it is not complete yet…so tell you later, but I was really impressed with their diagnosis system (check up methods) and treatment.

(Clinic of Russian Institute of Kibernatical Medicine, Russia, 117871, Moscow, Mikluho-Maklai Street, building number 16/10 Dr Viktor Gerasimovich, 007(095)3367900, info@cybermed.ru, www.cybermed.ru)."

Strokes

MR UPPAL mentioned strokes which are just as likely to affect women as men and in middle age, not just in old age. GP DR RICHARD HART says: *"My advice to avoid having a stroke is to eat well, sleep well, only drink in moderation and do not smoke".* (Ladies, is this starting to sound familiar? Whatever else you do in life, please do not smoke. It is the one thing that all the medical experts agree is truly dangerous for your health and it is certainly bad for your looks.)

Here is another word of warning regarding strokes. Consultant Gynaecologist and Obstetrician MR MICHAEL BOWEN (from whom we will be hearing later in this chapter) says *"do not take the Pill if you get focal migraines. There is already a risk that focal migraines can lead to a stroke. Taking the Pill definitely increases your risk of getting thrombosis and therefore of having a stroke. The longer you take the Pill and the more oestrogen that is in your Pill, the higher the risk. If you develop focal migraines while you are on the Pill, consult your doctor immediately and think about alternative contraception".*

Diabetes

MR UPPAL also mentioned diabetes which does, of course affect women as well as men. Even if you have never had it in youth and middle age you can get it in later life if you do not take care of your nutrition and lifestyle.

Opposite is a report on this unpleasant disease from health and beauty expert SIDRA SHAUKAT (www.sidrashaukat.biz), author of *Natural Beauty* (Chrysalis Books) and *Regenerate Yourself Younger.*

PREVENT DIABETES, PREVENT AGEING

from Sidra Shaukat

Diabetes is a subject very close to my heart. Having lost my father prematurely to this chronic disease, I know from first hand experience how crippling and destructive it really is. I was shocked to read that more than a third of the population born in 2000 will get diabetes. Type 2 diabetes, the type that typically arises from overeating and a sedentary lifestyle, accounts for more than 90% of diabetes cases.

If diagnosed with diabetes at age 40, men will lose 11.6 years of life and women will lose 14.3 years of life as a result of the disease. However, there are simple solutions that will prevent and even cure Type 2 diabetes. By controlling excess carbohydrate consumption and exercising, the body has to normalise its blood sugar levels.

Unfortunately, many are offered a drug solution such as insulin injections for a disease that can be prevented. Making changes in your life will help to optimise your insulin levels. Blood sugar is only the symptom in most diabetics so the real challenge is to control your insulin levels. Once the insulin levels are stabilised it is common for the blood sugar to come back to normal levels.

Exercise helps to combat insulin resistance by increasing the sensitivity of insulin receptors so the insulin that is present works effectively. Regular daily exercise can be as simple as a brisk walk for 30 minutes, an invigorating lunch-time swim or playing with children in the evening. Do whatever you love doing, but get active!

Exercise will not only make your insulin work harder, but it will also reduce your body fat. It has been shown that lean mammals live longer. Eating less produces fewer chemical by-products, known as free radicals, which can damage cells but leanness may also play a role in promoting longevity. Recent research could result in a new drug that would fight obesity, and related illnesses

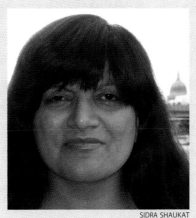

SIDRA SHAUKAT

like Type 2 diabetes, by blocking insulin receptors in fat tissue. The drug would need to be targeted to fat only, however, as a loss of insulin sensitivity through out the body results in Type 2 diabetes.

It appears that leanness is a key contributor to a long life, with insulin being the main reason. If you can understand insulin's role in health, you can prevent diabetes, ageing and disease.

You may have high insulin levels, if you have:

■ Excess weight
■ High Blood Pressure
■ High Blood Cholesterol
■ Diabetes

You can control your insulin levels by the following:

1 Increasing your activity and/or exercise, as mentioned above. Muscle works on the simple principle, if you don't use it, you lose it. A lean body will make you live longer and help your body use insulin efficiently.

2 Reducing your intake of refined simple carbohydrates such as white bread, cakes etc. These foods cause a surge in blood sugar, which acts as an alarm signal to the body to produce high insulin to stabilise it. Blood sugar drops very quickly

which makes you even more hungry and so the cycle is repeated. This results in a cycle of over-consumption that leads to weight gain.

3 Eat foods that keep blood sugar stable, such as oily fish, lean meat, porridge and high-fibre foods. Always try to eat protein and/or fat with carbohydrates to dampen the insulin response. Avoid eating unrefined carbohydrates on their own, as this will just cause the blood sugar highs and lows as discussed.

4 Avoid excess consumption of caffeine in tea, coffee, soft drinks. Caffeine also increases insulin levels, and if taken with sweets and carbs, you are doubling the dangerous effect of high blood sugar.

5 Try to prevent stress as much as possible. If you are highly stressed, make sure you take time out to relax, so the body can stabilise itself. Stress produces harmful hormonal reactions in the body, which also cause high insulin levels, so the cycles above continue.

You may be wondering why a simple thing like sugar can be the cause of so much disease. I used to think this as well, because as a child, I loved eating sweets as a reward for being a "good girl". The immediate reaction is that sugar tastes nice and sweet, so it must be good.

However, you have only to see how sticky it becomes, especially when it becomes caramel or toffee. This is why it is so toxic in the body. It literally sticks to proteins and causes havoc to the cells in the body. High blood sugar is one of the most degenerative factors in disease and ageing. So the answer is simple, prevent high insulin levels by controlling your blood sugar and you will prevent diabetes, disease and ageing.

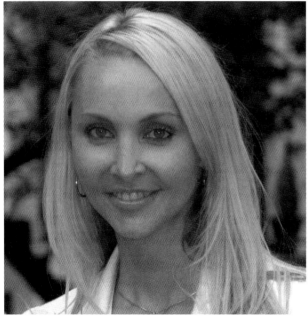

HEATHER BIRD

Anti-ageing

Then we come to the age-old (excuse the pun!) problem of ageing. Can we really live to be over a hundred with the zest of youth, as radical new technology suggests? Certainly we can feel and look MUCH better as we age nowadays. "American Beauty" HEATHER BIRD owns two popular anti-ageing clinics in London, HB Health of Harley Street and HB Health of 12 Beauchamp Place, SW3 1NZ, phone 020 7838 0765, is on the board of directors of the World Academy of Anti-Ageing Medicine (WAAAM) and sponsors and organises the Anti-Ageing Conference London (AACL). HEATHER says:

"I consider it my mission to work toward making the life enhancing medical breakthroughs of anti-ageing medical science available world-wide and to help people realise the full potential of their lives by promoting optimal health and wellness. At my clinics we focus on health as the key to beauty and quality of life. We work both internally and externally to take control of the ageing process and promote wellbeing.

Anti-Ageing is so much more than fighting wrinkles and looking younger. It is about feeling younger and functioning younger. Anti-Ageing medicine is a paradigm for proactive, preventative health care. It promotes not only living longer but also living better and healthier. Many of the physical and mental disabilities associated with normal ageing are caused by physiological dysfunctions that, in many cases, can be altered

by appropriate medical intervention based on the application of advanced scientific and medical technologies.

I am committed to advancing the cause of Anti-Ageing Medicine and helping it become a better established medical speciality in Britain and throughout Europe for the benefit of everyone."

DR LUCY GLANCEY, MRCS (Grove Clinic, Grove Farm, Grove Hill, Langham, Essex, CO4 5PJ, phone 0870 458 5483, www.glanceymedical.co.uk) is a member of the Royal College of Surgeons and the British Association of Cosmetic Doctors and is another well respected anti-ageing expert. TV favourite DR GLANCEY reports:

"The best way of fighting ageing is by good diet and dietary supplements; for instance papaya is supposed to be the new wonder food for anti-ageing. At the present time there is no good evidence to justify prescribing hormones as a preventative measure to counteract ageing and giving too many hormones can lead to cancer. Sooner or later, however, the drug companies may come up with hormone treatment which is effective and not harmful. At the moment lots of ladies in their thirties and forties who work in the City and other male dominated work areas are rubbing Testosterone cream into their inner arms and thighs to increase their energy and libido."

The menopause

These creams are also popular with menopausal women but a cream applied to the skin is obviously much less potent than a pill taken orally. There are several "natural HRT" pills on the market and then there is HRT itself. This is the big debate if you are menopausal or pre-menopausal: to HRT or not to HRT, that is the question. Of course women want to know how the menopause will affect them and what is the best way for them personally to get through this traditionally tricky period in life.

Fitness expert ANGELA BEST, ex wife of football hero GEORGE and mother of young gun CALLUM has written a very comprehensive book on the menopause called *Change for the Best: A Practical Guide to the Menopause* (Warner Books) which also contains valuable anti ageing advice. ANGELA advocates natural aids such as rubbing wild yam cream onto your skin and *"eating to control your hormones"*. For instance soy beans are apparently excellent and must be eaten for the rest of our lives once we reach the big five oh and a healthy diet of fruit, vegetables and fish will have a hormone regulating effect and keep us healthier and disease free for longer.

Here is a very comprehensive report on the menopause, including on HRT, from Consultant Gynaecologist and Obstetrician MR MICHAEL BOWEN, FRCS, MRCOG, MRCP (The Hospital of St John's and St Elizabeth's, Grove End Road, London, NW8, phone 020 7467 8471):

THE MENOPAUSE AND HRT
from Mr Michael Bowen, FRCS, MRCOG, MRCP

The average woman has a menopause around the age of 50. It is usually defined as the time when her periods stop, but prior to this some women may experience other symptoms such as hot flushes, difficulty in sleeping, restlessness, night sweats, depression, mood swings, tiredness, headaches and irregular periods. This is sometimes referred to as the perimenopausal period and is caused by the gradual decline in the production of the hormone oestrogen by the ovaries.

Throughout a woman's reproductive life the pituitary gland at the base of the brain produces two hormones: luteinising hormone (LH) and follicle stimulating hormone (FSH). These hormones enter the blood circulation and stimulate the ovaries to produce oestrogen. When enough oestrogen is produced by the ovaries, the pituitary gland detects this and slows down the production of FSH and LH. Conversely, if oestrogen levels are low then the levels of FSH and LH rise in an attempt to stimulate the ovaries more. Around the time of the menopause the ovaries lose their ability to produce oestrogen and, as a result, the pituitary gland increases production of FSH and LH in a response to the low oestrogen levels and in an attempt to drive the ovaries harder.

When you visit the doctor, the doctor may suggest taking a blood test which will confirm the menopause and it does this by showing a raised level of the hormones FSH and LH in your bloodstream. The menopause has become of interest relatively recently and this is only because men and woman were never expected to live much beyond the age of 50 in the "old days".

If you speak to 20 different women about their experience of the menopause they will give you 20 different answers and this tells us that the signs and symptoms can be very much an individual thing. Some women will report experiencing irregular periods and others will complain of all the possible symptoms.

Hot Flushes
The symptoms that women experience going through the menopause vary dramatically. Some will experience some hot flushes or they may find that they sweat a great deal, particularly at night, and become flushed. These attacks tend to occur at the start of the menopause and improve with time. They can occur several times an hour and frequently throughout the day, but usually last no more than three to six minutes.

Hot flushes may be extremely debilitating; some women have difficulty sleeping or falling asleep and often complain that they wake up at night dripping in sweat. This can be so severe that some women describe having to change their night clothes and bed sheets. The best treatment for these symptoms is oestrogen but there are alternatives which can help you cope.

Mood Changes
Mood swings, tiredness, headaches or even depression can be associated with the menopause. Many women describe the menopause as a dramatic change in their lives. Some experience a loss of confidence; some complain that their memory deteriorates and that they have less patience with people. This can create difficulties for a woman's family but equally the family may create difficulties for her! HRT may help with these symptoms but one should be mindful that "Mum's anger and explosion at a given event" might be rational, reasonable and commendable.

Skin can lose some of its integrity and become thinner, causing dryness. This occurs as a result of the reduction in oestrogens. The vagina in particular may not produce as much lubrication as it did before and this, coupled with oestrogen deficiency, may cause cracks and sores to appear in the vagina which can not only make sexual intercourse extremely uncomfortable it can cause discomfort at rest.

In conjunction with this, some women may find a change in libido where they are less interested in sex and it has been reported that orgasms or climax can become less intense. The lack of oestrogen can also affect the urinary system and part of the bladder may lose its integrity and become more sensitive. The result of this is that women may feel as if they have a bladder infection and want to pass urine more frequently.

Thinning of the Bones or Osteoporosis
One of the most important effects of the menopause is that it may cause thinning of the bones or osteoporosis. This loss of bone substance or thinning of the bones means that they are more prone to fractures and breaks. This may become apparent when they fall over and sustain a fracture, whereas at one time they would just develop some bruising. In extreme circumstances they may develop a pathological fracture where a bone may break even though it has been subject to only the normal day-to-day activities. This is particularly prominent where the bones in the vertebra or the backbone may fracture and collapse which can give women an abnormal curvature to the spine, sometimes referred to as a dowager's hump, and cause shrinking in height.

One of the areas where there has been great debate has been the effects of HRT on the cardiovascular system and what effects the menopause has on heart disease and strokes. It is noticeable that after the menopause a woman's risk of heart disease and strokes starts to rise in the same way as it does throughout a man's life. There has been speculation that HRT and delaying menopausal effects may change this risk. This is an exceptionally confusing area where the evidence of a dramatic effect one way or the other has been absent.

There is no doubt that in some women the symptoms of menopause are exceptionally disabling and those women will often seek some solution. The commonest form of treatment is hormone replacement therapy and this involves giving a small dose of oestrogen to replace the natural oestrogens a woman would have before the menopause. Oestrogen on its own can cause uterine disease so it is necessary to have some progestogens in addition to the oestrogen to protect the uterus from developing uterine cancers in the future. Naturally, if they have had a hysterectomy and their uterus removed then the progestogens are not necessary.

HRT has been shown to be effective in relieving hot flushes and vaginal dryness and some woman have reported a general improvement in their sense of well being. However, HRT is not a panacea and may have little effect on mood changes or behaviour as sometimes this is due to external factors that are unrelated to the menopause.

There is great debate about how long HRT should be taken for and some women may just take it for a short time of say six months to a year, purely to relieve their symptoms. Essentially, it does not matter how oestrogen enters your system. The commonest way to take it is in tablet form but other women may prefer to use skin patches, where it is absorbed through the skin, or an implant where it is implanted under the skin with local anaesthetic and will release the hormone over a period of time. Other forms of administering HRT include a form of gel that can be rubbed into the skin or a nasal spray.

HRT does not have any side effects in the majority of women and it is merely replacing the oestrogens that they would normally have. There are some women who may find it inconvenient experiencing periods again and others may report side effects such as nausea, breast tenderness, weight gain and fluid retention. These symptoms should settle down in the first few months of treatment but if they don't, it is possible to change the type of HRT you are taking or the way it is delivered to see if this makes a difference. It is worth visiting your GP or gynaecologist to discuss this.

The main risk of HRT is the development of breast cancers. On balance, women taking HRT live longer than those women who do not take it. The story of breast cancer and HRT is confusing. One study in 1997 looked at 1,000 European women who did not take hormone replacement therapy and found that 45 of them would develop a breast cancer during the time of the study. If these same women were to take HRT for five years there would be two extra women amongst the 1,000 who would develop breast cancer over five years. If they were to take HRT for ten years then there would be an extra six amongst them and for 15 years there would be an extra 12 women in the group who would develop breast cancer compared with those not taking it, that is:

- 1,000 women DO NOT take HRT, 45 will develop breast cancer
- 1,000 women take HRT for five years 47 will develop breast cancer
- 1,000 women take HRT for ten years 51 will develop breast cancer
- 1,000 women take HRT for 15 years 57 will develop breast cancer

Since most women take HRT for only a short time to control the menopausal symptoms, this risk is clearly very low.

This really can be quite complex for women who have had breast cancer or who have a family history of breast cancer. However, there are very few women where there is an absolute contraindication for taking hormone replacement therapy. It is stressed that women who are taking HRT should attend regular breast-screenings and perform self-examination.

There have been concerns about thromboembolic disorders and developing blood clots in the veins, (particularly of the legs) whilst taking HRT. The risk appears to be at its highest in the first year of taking it and then falls.

Women with a family history of thrombosis or a history of a previous thrombotic episode may need to have some special blood tests to see if there is a genetic predisposition to developing blood clots before deciding on HRT.

There are few absolute contraindications to HRT and very often the extra information will help identify the risks for a specific individual with a particular medical background or family history.

A woman has to look at the risks specifically for her taking HRT based on her history. It is important that she should be able to weigh up the pros and the cons and to decide for herself whether HRT is the right option. I must stress there is no absolute rule on any of these things and it is very much a matter of personal choice.

There are other ways of actually relieving some of the symptoms of the menopause and in particular it is possible to use oestrogens topically. This is particularly effective when treating vaginal dryness and if oestrogen creams or pessaries are used then there is very little systemic absorption, i.e. oestrogen entering the blood stream, reducing the risk of breast cancer or thromboembolic diseases.

Taking HRT after the natural menopause remains controversial; the large number of studies and amount of information does not necessarily give a consistent message and understandably causes some degree of confusion.

United States Women's Health Initiative Study

One notable study which caused wide scale concern was the United States Women's Health Initiative study. This is a study that looked at 16,000 healthy postmenopausal women. Half the women were taking hormone replacement therapy and the other half were taking a placebo (a tablet which they thought was hormone replacement therapy).

The women taking hormone replacement therapy were taking conjugated equine oestrogens with medroxyprogesterone [oestrogen from pregnant mare's urine and a particular type of progesterone which is an HRT combination not widely used in the UK].

This study was supposed to run for eight and a half years but it was stopped just after five years because women in the group who received hormone replacement therapy showed an increase in the incidence of breast cancer and overall there were concerns that the hormone replacement therapy was doing more harm than good. In particular, there appeared to be an increase in the risk of coronary heart disease, stroke and pulmonary embolism. However, there appeared to be some benefits also and there was a reduction in the number of women having hip fractures and colorectal cancer.

One of the problems with the way the study was reported is that it looked at hazard ratios rather than absolute numbers and the percentage of relative risk suggested there was a 26% increase in breast cancer, a 29% increase in heart disease, a 40% increase in strokes and a 213 % increase in the risk of pulmonary embolism. This caused alarm but was a misleading way of representing the results because in essence, with hormone replacement therapy, any percentage increase is of a small risk in the first place. For example, you might have a 200% increase in the risk of being struck

MR MICHAEL BOWEN

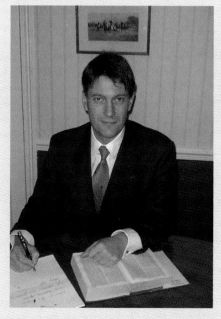

by lightning if you are standing under a tree, however the risk of being struck by lightning is incredibly small anyway.

When the absolute risks for 10,000 women taking HRT each year was looked at, it demonstrated that out of the 10,000 women there were an extra eight cases of breast cancer, an extra seven heart attacks, eight strokes and eight pulmonary emboli with a reduction in five hip fractures and six bowel cancers. This is out of 10,000 women so the overall results that you can see are negligible. At the same time there was a study in the United Kingdom of women taking oral oestradiol with norethisterone, which is a much more usual combination of HRT in the UK. This was looking at 100 post-menopausal women who had actually had a heart attack and the early results had shown no increase in the risk of having another heart attack.

However, as a result of the United States study, advice was given that women should not be given continuous combined hormone replacement therapy solely for the prevention of cardiovascular disease, should use alternative proven methods of improving their cardiovascular risk such as lipid-lowering drugs and antihypertensives and improve their lifestyle such as stopping smoking and losing weight.

For the women who were taking Premique, which was similar to hormone replacement therapy taken in the American study, in the Women's Health initiative, they were advised that if they wished to continue, stop or change to another regime, they should also be told that there is no data on the long-term safety for cardiovascular risk with any other alternative regime. The conclusion of this study suggested that unopposed oestrogen may be a safer option but this is only feasible for women who have had a hysterectomy as the risk if you are not taking progestogen with the oestrogens is that you might develop an endometrial cancer. The Women's Health Initiative did confirm that hormone replacement therapy prevents osteoporotic hip fractures and reduces the risk of colorectal cancer but the earlier claims about an improvement in cardiovascular disease could not be substanti-

ated. One of the criticisms of the study is that it did not evaluate the effects of hormone replacement therapy on the symptoms of quality of life and for many women these are important considerations and the major reasons for them continuing with hormone replacement therapy.

Oestrogen still remains the treatment of choice for hot flushes and is extremely effective. It is however known that smaller doses of hormone replacement therapy are as effective in controlling symptoms and preserving bone as higher doses. Venous thrombosis and developing clots in the veins is rare but can be a potentially catastrophic complication of taking HRT. It is important to actually be aware of your family history and if you are at risk, HRT may not be the right option for you.

It is important to appreciate why you are taking hormone replacement therapy and if it is for specific treatment of symptoms such as vaginal soreness, sometimes known as senile vaginitis, then topical oestrogen treatments are just as effective and do not have the same side effects as taking the tablets.

The important hormone to take for hormone replacement therapy is oestrogen; however, as I have previously mentioned if you have a uterus in place it is important to take some progestogens. However, it is possible to actually look at varying the dose of progestogen and taking them in alternative combinations. This effect can be manipulated with tablets so that you may just have a vaginal bleed once every three months rather than once a month. Alternatively the progestogens may be delivered locally to the uterus by using a progestogen-impregnated intrauterine contraceptive device where, similar to using oestrogen cream, progestogen just acts locally on the uterine lining and very little is absorbed into the system.

Weight gain is probably one of the great concerns of women taking hormone replacement therapy and is a serious concern for many patients. There is very little evidence to suggest that hormone replacement therapy is responsible for large weight gain; however if you recognise it as the increase in maturity, you can become less active and the fat distribution tends to be around the waist rather than around the hips and bottom. Some women like taking HRT and it improves their well-being. There is nothing to say you cannot take HRT long-term; however you should be aware of the risks and be making an informed choice as to whether this is the right option for you.

One Million Women Study

With regard to breast cancer, another study which caused a sensation was the breast cancer and hormone replacement therapy in the One Million Women study. This study looked at one million women and was set up to investigate the effects of specific types of hormone replacement therapy on the incidence and the risk of breast cancer. The study was over five years and looked at women attending a breast screening clinic and asked them about their hormone replacement therapy habits. Of those attending the breast screening clinic, half of them had used hormone replacement therapy and current users of hormone replacement therapy were more likely than those who had never used it to develop breast cancer and die from it.

Past users of hormone replacement therapy were not at increased risk of developing the disease or dying from it. This incidence was significantly increased for women using only oestrogen by factor of 1.3, those using oestrogen and progestogen by a factor of 2 and those using tibolone by a factor of 1.45. Obviously, those women using a combined preparation of oestrogen and progestogen have the greatest risk of developing breast cancer.

The specific type of oestrogens and progestogens, their doses or the way they were prescribed did not appear to make much difference.

The risks of breast cancer were significantly increased for those using oral rather than transdermal and implanted oestrogen-only formulations. Of the current users who are using hormone replacement therapy, the risk of breast cancer increases with the increase in total duration of use. So after ten years of using hormone replacement therapy post-menopause, there are an additional five breast cancers per one thousand using oestrogen alone and 19 for those using oestrogen and progestogen combinations.

This led to the report that HRT over the past decade has resulted in an estimated 20,000 extra breast cancers, with 15,000 of those associated with oestrogen and progestogen. The big question is: is HRT going to kill you? But it is not possible to reliably estimate what the extra deaths would be.

Another cancer blow to HRT: Swedish study shows higher risk to breast tumour survivors

A study performed in Sweden demonstrated there is a higher risk for those women who survive breast cancer. Here, they looked at the women's medical histories for just over two of the five years originally planned; the results suggested that risk of recurrence was more than three times higher for those on HRT compared with those not taking HRT.

However, the numbers of women studied were relatively small (174)

Twenty-six of the 174 women on HRT who reported a recurrence or a new case of breast cancer compared with seven of the 171 who were not taking HRT. Other studies have suggested that this difference may not be so significant. Nevertheless, this trial caused some degree of alarm and had to be stopped because of concern about causing harm to the patients in the trial.

If you are confused, you would be no different from your doctor. The suggestion is that the minimum effective dose of HRT should be used for the shortest duration to combat menopausal symptoms. These decisions have been criticised for exaggerating the dangers of HRT and for leaving women with little official guidance on effective alternatives to combating menopause or preventing osteoporosis. Companies selling herbal and vitamin supplements are seeking to fill that gap.

It is not surprising that there is such a large interest in herbal and vitamin supplements which may be an alternative for patients not wishing to expose themselves to these dangers. However one should bear in mind that we only know about the risks of conventional HRT because they have been subjected to large scale studies whereas many other alternative medications have not been formally evaluated.

So now you know just about all there is to know about this important time in a woman's life and the possible therapy, thanks to MR BOWEN. Although the jury's not yet out on HRT, you can make an informed choice, preferably after also consulting your GP and/or gynaecologist. There certainly are a great deal of alternative pills for the menopause on the shelves of pharmacies and supermarkets but some of them allegedly give users unpleasant side effects.

If you live in the US or are happy to wait for overseas products to arrive, EMERITA MENOPAUSE SOLUTIONS manufactured by TRANSITIONS FOR HEALTH INC. (Portland, OR 97205 USA), phone 1-800 455 5182, www.emerita.com) have a wide range of homeopathic products.

On the HRT plus front, one of my friend's mothers has been happily "on it" for 17 years without any noticeable side effects and in fact gets very moody if she goes off it for any length of time and some mature beauties such as KATE O'MARA swear by it. Only time will tell whether the benefits outweigh the risks.

Taste

5
FOOD FOR THOUGHT
THE BRAIN, THE MIND, THE SOUL

I is generally accepted that fish is good brain food. Sadly, however, fish is not sensually pleasurable on the smell front so you may prefer to eat your fresh fish when dining out in winter and open the windows when cooking fish at home in summer. Smoked fish will not stink out your home and oily fish is now considered excellent for the skin so load up the fridge with smoked salmon immediately and the bathroom cupboard with Gold Spot for your breath!

Fish

Overleaf there is a fantastic three course menu featuring fish created by restaurateur and celebrity TV Chef BRIAN TURNER, CBE of BRIAN TURNER MAYFAIR (Millennium Hotel, Grosvenor Square, London W1K 2HP, phone 020 7596 3444) and TURNER'S GRILL (The Copthorne Hotel, Slough, Windsor, Berks, phone 01753 607 352).

Brian trained at SIMPSON'S IN THE STRAND and THE SAVOY GRILL and worked at CLARIDGE'S and THE CAPITAL HOTEL where he and RICHARD SHEPHERD earned a prized MICHELIN STAR. He was for many years resident chef on GRANADA'S *This Morning* before moving to the BBC for his own series, *Anything You Can Cook* and is a star of *Ready Steady Cook*. In 2002 he was honoured with a CBE for his services to tourism and training in the catering industry.

As you can see, this marvellous menu is also completely wheat and dairy free so it is extra healthy. This being the case you can afford to have lots of delicious tatties on the side if you feel like it!

Coffee

Coffee can stimulate the brain for a short while and alcohol will dull your senses but an Irish Coffee every now and then is a truly sensual pleasure, especially when shared. As is *"coppa dell'amicizia"* from the Italian Alps. ALBERTO PAGANO, owner of RISTORANTE CAPPUCCETTO (8/9 Moor Street, London W1, phone 020 7437 9472, www.alcappuccetto.co.uk) who makes the best *"coppa dell'amicizia"* tells me that this delicious after dinner drink is a mixture of hot coffee, grappa, orange peel, Cointreau and *other ingredients*. It is served in a carved mahogany kettle for two, four or six to share. Simply delicious!

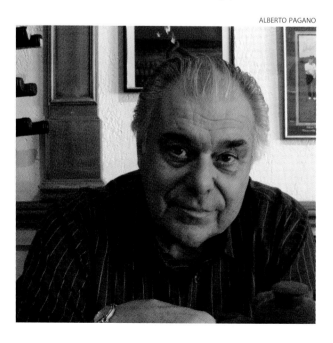

ALBERTO PAGANO

THREE COURSE FISH MENU

by Restaurateur and Celebrity TV Chef, Brian Turner CBE

Course one: Starter

Cushions of Whitby/local smoked salmon with cockle and parsley dressing   *Serves 4*

INGREDIENTS

CUSHIONS OF SALMON

4 large slices smoked salmon
6 oz fresh cooked salmon
2 tbsp mayonnaise
2 finely chopped shallots
2 tbsp chopped chives
1 tbsp vinaigrette
1 tbsp chopped spring onions
salt & pepper

COCKLE DRESSING

4 oz cooked cockles
½ tsp Dijon mustard
1 tbsp white wine vinegar
4 tbsp olive oil
2 tbsp chopped parsley
½ clove crushed garlic
1 tbsp tomato concasse
salt & pepper

METHOD

1 Lay one slice of smoked salmon on cling film.
2 Flake salmon into a bowl, do not break up too much.
3 Add mayonnaise, shallots, chives, vinaigrette and spring onion, season and allow to stand for ten minutes.
4 Spoon a quarter of the mix onto centre of smoked salmon.
5 Pull in sides of smoked salmon then use cling film to pull in and seal gently into ball shape.
6 Push into 2-inch ring, joins uppermost – put into fridge to chill.
7 Make sauce by mixing cockles and mustard.
8 Add white wine vinegar, stir, add oil and parsley, garlic and tomato and mix in.
9 Season and put to one side.
10 Carefully take out salmon, unwrap and turn over onto a plate.
11 Pour sauce around, brush salmon with oil and serve.

Course two: Main course

Brill on sweet peppers and garlic   *Serves 4*

INGREDIENTS

4 x 5 oz brill fillet (off bone)
2 finely chopped shallots
1 glass white wine
½ pt fish stock
1 tbsp olive oil

2 sweet red peppers
8 cloves garlic
2 tbsp chopped chives
salt & pepper

METHOD

1 Put the brill in tray on chopped shallots add white wine and fish stock.
2 Cover with greaseproof paper.
3 Put in the oven 180°c and bake until just cooked.
4 Remove from the oven and take out of tray, keep warm and covered.
5 Reduce stock to ¼ by volume.
6 Meanwhile warm olive oil.
7 Trim peppers, cut into ½ inch squares.
8 Add to oil and stew slowly.
9 Blanche garlic twice in water and refresh.
10 Add garlic to peppers and slowly cook out.
11 Add stock to peppers, reboil, add chives and season with salt and pepper.
12 Put brill on plate then carefully pour peppers over and around and serve.

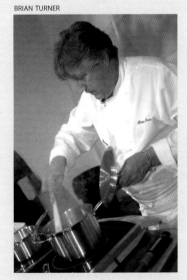

BRIAN TURNER

Course three: Dessert

Chilled melon soup with mint and raspberries   *Serves 4*

INGREDIENTS

1 Charentais melon
1 Ogen melon
150 g castor sugar
8 oz raspberries
1 tbsp chopped mint

METHOD

1 Halve and seed the melons.
2 Using a melon "baller" cut the flesh into ball shapes and put into fridge.
3 Scoop out the rest of the flesh and add to the sugar in a food processor.
4 Blitz and then put into an ice cream machine or, taking longer, put into a tray in the freezer.
5 Do not let the mixture freeze solid, use a whisk to mix the freezer version.
6 Put the melon balls and raspberries in a large chilled martini glass.
7 Mix the mint with the frozen soup and pour over the fruit to serve.

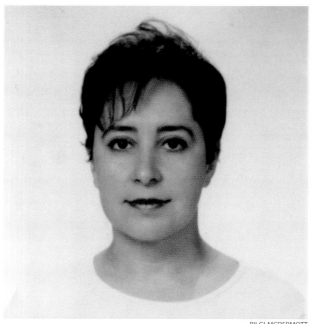

BILGI MCDERMOTT

Integrative psychotherapy

What about sustenance for your mind and your soul, your spirit? My advice to you is to enjoy the sensual pleasures inherent in the wonders of nature every day of your life and "don't sweat the small stuff"! If you have serious psychological, spiritual or emotional problems you will need to seek professional advice. It is quite acceptable to be "in therapy" in today's highly stressful world. After all there is no point in having a healthy body if your mind and spirit are unhealthy. My counsellor BILGI MCDERMOTT (phone 020 7381 9407, mobile 07747 876 294) who got me through the extreme emotional pain of my parents' deaths, is an "Integrative Psychotherapist". This is what BILGI has to say about this sort of therapy, which can help everyone and is becoming more and more available worldwide:

"Integrative Psychotherapy considers the importance of the whole person, paying attention to thoughts, feelings and somatic symptoms which cause distress. The counsellor/psychotherapist seeks to move beyond these painful symptoms to engage with you at the cause of your disturbance with the intention that you will gain a greater sense of well-being in your life and improve your capacity for flexibility, choice and change."

Depression

Issues which can be addressed through Integrative Psychotherapy include loss and bereavement, depression and anxiety, identity crisis, relationship difficulties and eating disorders. So do not just suffer debilitating emotional pain – get professional help; it is the healthy alternative to going on the dreaded PROZAC which can slow you down in many ways, including sexually.

We all strive more than anything to be happy in our lives and having a good laugh always lifts our mood. When CLINIQUE were developing their "HAPPY" range of fragrances they consulted John Morreall, PhD, a psychologist and President of Humorworks Seminars in Tampa, Florida who told the cosmetics company *"after you laugh, you get into a relaxed state. Your blood pressure and heart rate drop below normal, so you feel profoundly relaxed. Laughter also indirectly stimulates endorphins, the brain's natural painkillers"*. My advice to you is to try to cultivate happy people in both your private and professional lives and to help people who are not naturally happy for whatever reason by making them laugh. The healthier you are in your body, the better you will feel in your soul and the more capable you will be of getting through the inevitable horrid patches that life throws at all of us.

"I find shared laughter a most important element in any relationship."

Larry Adler – *Have I ever told you…*

Taste

6

CELLULITE &
FATTY TISSUES & ISSUES

ELLULITE is seriously "big stuff". As Fitness and Beauty Editor of HOT GOSSIP UK, I receive more mail about cellulite than any other subject, including boobs and wrinkles! The women of the world are obsessed with the orange peel effect and rightly so. I have seen girls of thirteen with cellulite, women of sixty and even men with what looks suspiciously like it. It is the modern (mostly) female ailment and I am convinced it is caused as much by lifestyle, preserved foods and stress as by fatness and hormones. In fact the slimmest, fittest ladies can have small patches of cellulite on their thighs, bums and tums and I have even seen professional athletes with the problem. There is only one type of build that does not seem cellulite prone and that is the wider-torsoed lady with long, slim arms and legs. For the rest of us I am afraid we just have to accept that we may one day get cellulite even if we do not have it now and we will need to operate a strict "prevention and cure" plan from an early age.

SO WHAT EXACTLY IS CELLULITE ANYWAY?

Beauty expert SIDRA SHAUKAT, author of *Natural Beauty*
and creator of "Buff's IncrEdible Edibles" range of 100% natural treatments, reports:

The current ideal for viewing the female and male body as youthful which entails the presence of well defined muscles and very little body fat has led to the development of a new medical "disease" – cellulite. Cellulite is a physiological condition that is caused by excess fatty tissue retention in the so called sub-dermal layer (that is just under the skin). In this tissue layer the fat cells are divided by fibrous strands into little compartments much like cells in a honey comb. If you imagine an overfilled honey comb with the honey causing each compartment to bulge that is how excess fat creates the orange skin appearance which women hate so much.

The reason why I say women is because it really is an oestrogen driven process. Almost all women except those that are extremely thin will store fat in their buttocks and thighs. The more fat stored the more apparent the cellulite becomes. Men anatomically have less subcutaneous fat and thicker skin which makes cellulite rare. Cellulite may be divided into primary cellulite which results from the accumulation of extra fat into the fat cells and secondary cellulite which results from ageing and from increased laxity of the skin and therefore relaxation of the walls of the fat cells.

You can determine the extent of cellulite by pinching the skin of the thigh between both hands (mattress phenomenon). Cellulite appears as a dimpling of the pinched skin and can be graded one to four according to the degree of surface irregularity. In the best scenario cellulite is visible only with pinching, as occurs in very thin women and in the worst cases will not only be clearly visible but the skin surface will have an uneven almost pebble stone texture to touch.

The same foods and drinks that lead to bad health can also exacerbate cellulite: TV dinners, sodas, coffee and tea and alcohol (sorry!) So please cut out or moderate all those naughty things in your diet. On the other hand all fresh foods and particularly papaya, mangoes and pineapple will allegedly ward off the dreaded dimpled effect.

Cellulite treatments

You may be able to nip incipient cellulite in the bud by using any of a vast array of anti cellulite creams currently available; CLARINS "Total Body Lift" is one of the most popular and effective, for instance. DR PATRICK BOWLER MS.BS, LRCP, MRCS, DRCOG is the chairman and co-founder (with DR RITA RAKUS) of the British Association of Cosmetic Doctors and knows everything there is to know about the dreaded orange peel condition. His "Vitage Antioxidant Body Refining Gel" is the latest "miracle product" to try (available from DR BOWLER at The Courthouse Clinic, 30B Wimpole Street, London, W1, phone 0870 850 3456).

Mesotherapy

However if your cellulite is particularly stubborn and/or you are older or carrying excess weight, you may need to bring out the big guns to fight it. MESOTHERAPY is a brilliant anti-cellulite treatment involving injections and SISTER MALTI O'MAHONY, founder of the world famous BOSTON CLINIC has recently pioneered a new treatment called MESO-MESH for more mature gals who need saggy skin plumped up at the same time. Overleaf SISTER O'MAHONY (THE BOSTON CLINIC and BOSTON AESTHETICS CLINIC, 41 and 63A Moscow Road, Bayswater, W2 4JS, phone 020 7229 3904/020 7229 8890, www.boston-clinic.co.uk, www.bostonaestheticsclinic.co.uk) tells us even more about cellulite and her treatments for it.

Endermologie

If you cannot stand needles, another excellent anti-cellulite treatment which is quite painless and extremely relaxing is ENDERMOLOGIE which involves firm machine massage whilst wearing a light "all in one" body suit. Cosmetic doctor DR LUCY GLANCEY is an authority on cellulite and has had great success with Endermologie. In the panel below she talks about Endermologie and the prevention of cellulite.

ENDERMOLOGIE

from Dr Lucy Glancey

Endermologie is a suction massage device originating from France and then introduced to the United States in 1991. The theory behind its mechanism of action is that it pulls the patients skin up into a set of rollers under a low pressure vacuum. The rolling motion and the pressure difference are thought to stretch the connective tissue under the skin which is responsible for the formation of the typical cellulite (orange peel) appearance. This also improves the lymphatic flow. There have been a number of different studies reporting a success rate of this treatment, ranging from 30% to 50%, but all studies point towards the fact that using longer treatment regimens is the best way to improve the cellulite reduction effect of Endermologie. Another way is to begin treatment after liposuction. When lipo-suction is combined with Endermologie it is much easier to contour the fat because it has already been damaged during the liposuction process so it can be readily moulded into a desired new shape.

In addition, multiple studies with Endermologie have shown that younger patients respond best to Endermologie because they have not yet developed advanced cellulite.

How to prevent cellulite. It must be remembered that there is a significant hereditary factor when it comes to cellulite. There are some women that are very thin, but never the less still have cellulite. However, as the amount of subcutaneous fat determines the degree of cellulite, a sensible diet has to be followed in order to keep this amount of fat under control.

It is important that the diet regime is followed over long periods of time to maintain a stable weight and avoid yo-yo dieting. This type of crash diet to lose a large amount of weight in a certain time is undesirable because it does not allow the excess skin that had previously been stretched over the fatty areas to shrink back and therefore the dieter may end up with unsightly areas of loose skin.

Physical exercise is important as it helps to convert the fatty tissue into energy which leads to decrease in the excess fat and hence cellulite. On the other hand it also helps to increase the muscle bulk which, in contrast to the fatty tissue which accumulates in large lumps, grows in a more uniform and aesthetically pleasing manner.

MESO-MESH

from Sister Malti O'Mahony

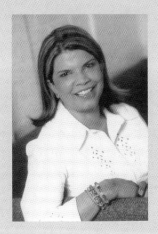

Contrary to popular belief, cellulite is not caused by excess weight. Typically (although not exclusively) a female problem, it can affect women of all ages and sizes. In women, fat cells on the lower part of the body store fat six times more readily than those on the upper body. They also release them six times less readily.

You can check to see if you have cellulite by pinching the skin around your upper thigh. If it looks a bit lumpy, you probably have it. And if you have cellulite, you are definitely not alone. According to recent research, 95% of women suffer from cellulite.

The problem only becomes worse with time. Gradually, the lumpy orange-peel effect of cellulite will be more pronounced on the hips, abdomen, thighs and buttocks. A more sedentary lifestyle and unbalanced diet contribute further to the development of cellulite and the appearance of localised rolls of fat.

What is cellulite?

Cellulite is the development of degraded fatty tissue that frequently contains water. This disorder results from one or several factors such as poor arterial or venous circulation, hormonal disturbances and problems with lymphatic drainage. Cellulite is due to the excessive storage of fat in the adipocytes. By becoming heavily laden with lipids, the adipocytes swell and become hypertrophic, sometimes to a high degree. The compression of the blood and lymph vessels by these fatty masses induces poor drainage of the water and stagnation of the toxins in the tissues. The resulting oedema and degeneration of the fibres of the connective tissue lead to the typical irregular stippled appearance of the skin known as "orange skin".

Cellulite is frequently associated with circulation problems. The adipocytes, swollen by an excessive accumulation of fat exert pressure on the arterial venous and lymphatic networks which surround them.

What is mesotherapy?

Mesotherapy is a homeopathic-based medical treatment that has been practised for over thirty-five years in Europe. It was first discovered by an Italian doctor. The medicine used from mesotherapy is vitamin B1, a component of the vitamin B complex family, mixed with a local anaesthetic. This medicine is an extract of plants, vegetables and minerals. This does not pose any problem as they have no secondary effects on the body. These are adapted for use in an injection form. Tiny injections of this mixture are injected into the cellulite or fatty tissue to improve circulation of lymphatic and venous drainage by increasing metabolism of the injected area.

Having performed their therapeutic task, the medicine is then broken down by the enzymes in the bloodstream and transported to the kidney to be removed as a waste body product via urine. Therefore, very little, if any medicine reaches the general circulation and in any case the level is so low that it has no effect on the rest of the body.

After initial consultation and assessment, the recommendation will be suggested for the set of treatments required. We recommend mesotherapy for all types of cellulite and fatty areas, including advanced cases

with steatoma (hard fatty tissue) which is the lumpy, sluggish, orange peel effect on the top of the thighs.

It also treats symptoms of cellulite such as heavy legs and thighs, saddles, love handles, upper arms, inner and outer thighs, poor circulation, toxin deposits, bad diet and lack of exercise.

The benefit of mesotherapy is that the symptoms of cellulite such as heavy or swollen legs rapidly disappear. In fact, heavy or swollen legs often feel better after the first couple of treatments.

Once the cellulite has gone, with a bit of patience and will power, good diet and routine exercise, it should be possible to ensure the cellulite of fat remains at bay.

Occasionally top-up treatment may be needed every three months. This is usually because of factors such as busy lifestyles, stress and pollution. The best way to avoid cellulite is to eat a healthy diet, drinking plenty of water, eating fresh fruit, vegetables and cutting down on wheat and dairy products.

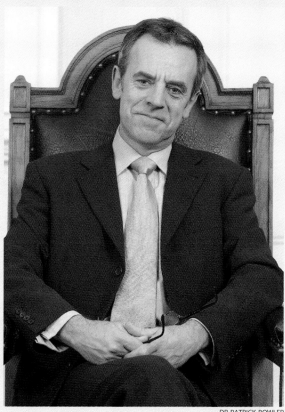

DR PATRICK BOWLER

TRI-ACTIVE
Three-Fold Action Fights Cellulite

Tri-active is the result of DEKA's new technology based on the combination of three different methods capable of restoring a normal balance to your skin. This treatment is designed to dramatically reduce the appearance of cellulite using a unique and painless **Dermodynamic** method: the combined action of a localised cooling system, rhythmic massage and deep laser stimulation. The deep massaging and stimulating action on the subcutaneous tissue allow toxin elimination and tissue oxygenation, thus creating a smoother appearance of the skin

- **Massage** A penetrating massage stimulates lymph drainage that provides a greater elasticity and flexibility to the skin
- **Cooling** Cryotherapy aids in cellulite reduction by reducing oedema and stimulating vascular activity in combination with the laser
- **Stimulation** The diode laser action deeply stimulates blood microcirculation within the veins and arteries while also increasing lymphatic capacity

Tri-active can also be used to enhance the results of liposuction. Each session lasts approximately twenty minutes and a course of twelve treatments is recommended for optimum results.

Tri-active

The most recent cellulite treatment to reach the UK from Italy is DEKA's TRI-ACTIVE machine, which is exclusive in this country to cosmetic doctor DR PATRICK BOWLER (THE COURT HOUSE CLINIC, 30B Wimpole Street, London, W1, phone 0870 850 3456). DR BOWLER believes the TRI-ACTIVE works on cellulite particularly well in younger patients. This brand new machine which is manufactured by medical giants CYNOSURE UK LTD (012628 522252, www.cynosure-laser.co.uk) looks just like a leggy Dalek but has proved very successful already. At the bottom left is the TRI-ACTIVE bumph.

The TRI-ACTIVE machine can also be used to smooth the skin after liposuction procedures (which we will come to in a later chapter) and is excellent for lifting the bum, an important consideration as we all want pert posteriors, do we not?

Lipostabil

The latest fat zapping treatment is LIPOSTABIL, also known as LIPODISSOLVE and, colloquially, as THE FLAB JAB! This is an amazing new treatment which actually gets rid of really stubborn small areas of fat that will not go away with diet or exercise, for instance double chins, jowls, bums, tums and knees. LIPOSTABIL can also be used on certain types and areas of cellulite. It is much less invasive than LIPOSUCTION and just involves injecting the product which then dissolves the fat.

At the time of writing LIPOSTABIL has not yet been passed by the MHRA, but it probably will be soon as it is already "legal" abroad. It will definitely be available in some London clinics, including the BOSTON CLINICS but you will need a doctor's prescription for it.

Practitioners will also insist upon a cholesterol test for safety before treating patients with LIPOSTABIL. Reading your cholesterol levels is a simple procedure involving a small prick in the finger and only takes two minutes. You can get it done free at your local Boots and it is not a bad idea to have the test anyway if you are middle aged, overweight or there is a history of high cholesterol in your family.

Taste

7

EXERCISE

Burn up your food and liquid intake and get those endorphins going with a spot of exercise, ladies. Endorphins are feel good hormones which the body produces when exercising: a natural and wonderful mood elevator. Even if you have a perfect figure and eat and drink sensibly you will feel much fitter, healthier and happier if you take at least a little gentle exercise. Don't you want that handsome waiter in your local Italian restaurant to say "you have a good *fisic* (physique), madam"? (Or even "miss" if you are looking particularly delectable!)

One thing that exercise is good for is your circulation and thus your skin and any incipient cellulite which may be lurking beneath the surface of the skin (or, God forbid, above it!) By the way if you have a tendency towards cramp you may need to exercise more and improve your circulation. Salt is supposed to help but too much is not good for you in general. In actual fact drinking Tonic Water is an "old wives' tale" which really works for cramp: try it.

Exercise will also keep you looking and feeling youthful. Opposite is an excerpt from health and beauty expert SIDRA SHAUKAT's new book *Regenerate Yourself Younger, The Scientific Proof for Preventing Disease and Ageing* (details from www.sidrashaukat.biz).

Once you have decided to embark upon a fitness regime you must decide what sort of exercise will be best for you personally. First up is the dreaded gym which is probably the easiest and most accessible way to exercise. Most gyms have music and/or TVs to watch while you are slaving away which makes it easier. Once you have sorted out your routine and know it, you can plug yourself in to the telly, talk on your mobile phone ("hands free", please, for health reasons) and even read the paper during seated exercises!

Here is all you need to know about training for ladies from NICK RETTER, Personal Trainer at my gym, ENERGIZE! (Hammersmith College, West London, phone 020 8748 9933, www.energizefitness.co.uk) where they have excellent LIFE FITNESS machines to exercise your every muscle.

"The advantages of gym training are achieving fitness and stamina, strength, overall looks and well-being and improving posture.

If you are aiming for cardiovascular fitness you should do some exercise which involves working your heart and lungs. This could be a treadmill, stepper, crosstrainer or bike. Spending 30 minutes three days a week will help keep your heart fit and will help you burn extra calories which will aid in weight loss if you are following a calorie controlled diet.

For muscle tone you should aim for 12–15 repetitions 2–3 times using a variety of machines which will give you a total body workout.

The areas that women are most interested in working on are usually their upper arms, stomachs, bottoms and thighs. The best exercise for the triceps (upper arms) is the Seated Triceps Extension, for the stomach the Abcradle, for the bottom and legs the Glut Machine, squats or lunges with free weights and for isolating the legs, the Abductor and Adductor for outer and inner thighs, leg extensions and leg curls for the fronts and backs of the thighs.

Do not eat a big meal for two hours before your training and try to eat something within two hours (maximum) afterwards to replace lost energy. You can drink water all the way through your routine and a carbohydrate drink if you are doing prolonged exercise (lasting more than an hour).

EXERCISE TO KEEP YOUR BODY YOUNG AND FIT

from Sidra Shaukat

There is nothing more ageing than carrying extra weight. Everyone who loses weight immediately claims to have more energy, vigour, looks and feels younger. Medical research recommends 30 minutes of exercise per day to maintain good health, 60 minutes per day to lose weight.

A trim waistline makes you look younger, so concentrate on exercises such as sit-ups and side stretches to work your obliques. As you get older, you need to add ten minutes to your workout because after 30, a decreasing metabolism results in muscle loss, which means we burn less calories. Yoga is a great anti-ageing exercise which gives a supple body and calm mind.

Regular gentle exercise is better for your body than heavy exercise. Exercise keeps muscles strong. It also increases blood supply to the brain keeping the mind active. Stretching increases flexibility and helps maintain co-ordination, reducing the risk of falling in old people.

Don't go overboard. Professor Axt from Germany, author of *On the Joy of Laziness*, advises,

"Waste half your free time. Just enjoy lazing around. People who would rather laze in a hammock instead of running a marathon or who take a midday nap instead of playing squash have a better chance of living into old age."

Exercise decreases blood sugar and improves the body's ability to use glucose for energy.

Exercise decreases the risk of developing diabetes and heart disease and helps to control blood pressure and maximises weight loss.

The most effective exercise routine is a combination of strength training (with an extra focus on mid-section), cardiovascular exercise (short, hard workouts) and stable blood sugar (keeps you from adding additional fat and makes it easier for the body to use body fat for fuel).

Use short, hard cardio workouts to increase metabolism

Cardio workouts can increase your metabolism, even hours after your workout, so you burn more calories whilst you sleep! Excess calories do not get stored as body fat because they are more likely to be used by your elevated metabolism. You also burn off some excess body fat.

Stabilise blood sugar

To effectively stabilise your blood sugar, you need to eat frequently, like every 2–3 hours. This gives your body only what it needs at that time. Your body burns calories 24 hours a day, so eating a few large meals creates sugar peaks and lows. Have

adequate nutrition by giving your body the fuel it needs: vegetables, fruits, nuts, berries, whole grains, and lean proteins (chicken, fish, lean beef, eggs, etc.). There is too much emphasis on how much fat is in food, or how "healthy" it is. Calories are the same no matter where they come from. Any extra calories become body fat.

Ask the professionals

Unfortunately, most people don't know enough about the human body, nutrition, or effective exercise. If you are not happy with your fitness you should consider getting the help of a qualified personal fitness professional, who can help you achieve your health and fitness goals effectively.

The strategies discussed in this article can help you take control of your metabolism, burn off that excess body fat and have you looking and feeling great! End result, a younger, fitter body.

You can do cardiovascular training every day but you should only do weight training three times a week. Work your whole body and incorporate cardiovascular fitness into your routine. Watch your calorie intake if you want to lose weight."

Do not overdo your training especially if you are working with weights: huge muscles are not sexy on a woman and you should not become obsessed with working out. As with so many health issues, moderation is the key. Gym gloves, available from most sports shops, are a must if you are using machines for your arm exercises; callused hands are extremely un-goddess like and will not feel sensually pleasurable to the touch!

If you enjoy going to classes, there are as many dance and fitness studios as there are gymnasiums nowadays and most gyms also run classes. AEROBICS and STEP classes are great

for building up stamina and becoming really fit and there are all sorts of BODY CONDITIONING classes available if you just want to tone and sculpt your body.

There are now more fitness videos than ever on the market so, if you prefer to exercise "in the comfort of your own home", invest in a few different ones to allay boredom and get going. But no slacking just because you are by yourself with no competition!

However if you are looking for a type of exercise which is more sensually pleasurable, you should try dance or at least dance-based fitness classes or videos. Dancing will help your posture and learning routines is great for both your brain and your self-confidence. Do not worry if you are not a natural twinkle toes like WAYNE SLEEP: you will still be getting some exercise and probably having fun too.

WHAT IS AEROBIC EXERCISE?

from Kardy Laguda

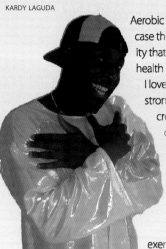

KARDY LAGUDA

Aerobic means "with oxygen" and if that is the **case then** we can walk, jog, run or do any activity **that** requires us to use oxygen in order for our **health** benefits to increase.

I love the thought of using music with a **strong** beat to move to and that is why I have **created** Kardy's Dance Aerobic Party workout which shows you simple steps that get you moving to a good strong beat.

You can do this kind of activity with friends and family and with any piece of music that makes you tap your feet or nod your head.

The idea behind movement related **exercise** programs is the element because **that** is what makes it a repeatable event and

with repetition comes familiarity and with that comes confidence which turns into more effort which transforms into results and all of this is encompassed around…you got it! – FUN!

Why do something that bores you witless if you can get the same results from something you like?

The frequency of such an activity has to be a minimum of three times a week but you must not overdo it in the initial stages. Avoid starting at 100% energy as your body may not be ready for this and what was fun may turn out to be quite traumatic.

The duration? Well, that is up to the individual or your expert but I will suggest that you listen to your body and if something does not feel right just tone it down or stop.

Most of all my message is clear: move to music that you love and smile, have fun!

In the panel above, dancer, choreographer and fitness expert KARDY LAGUDA (07860 468 222, www.solidsounduk.com), whose KARDY'S DANCE AEROBIC PARTY video is a perennial best-seller, talks about dance-based aerobics.

Ballroom dancing

Ballroom dancing is definitely sensually pleasurable and has become very popular recently. World Champion ballroom dancer and star of STRICTLY COME DANCING, PAUL KILLICK reports that more and more ladies and gentlemen are flocking to his DANCESPORT studio (57 Pont Street, London, SW1X 0BD, phone 020 7589 3071, www.paulkillick.com) to learn both ballroom and Latin American dance (which is really sexy and sensual).

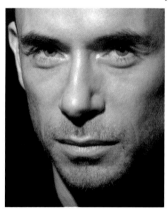

PAUL KILLICK

PAUL says *"Ballroom and Latin American dancing ignite the fire within us whatever age, culture or background. Cultivating a feeling of exhilaration, fitness, weight loss and social skills. Some of the benefits include:*

🏃 Exercising gently but still getting great results.

🏃 Achieving an aerobic workout without watching the clock!

🏃 Improving posture, keeping the body supple and preventing back problems later in life.

🏃 Gaining elegance, poise and grace.

🏃 And all important, Dance has the ability to arouse the passion and freedom of spirit within us all.

What is more you will have a jolly good time and make lots of new friends, some of whom might even be of the male variety!

Belly dancing

BELLY DANCING is another sensually pleasurable form of dance which is also great for our pelvic floors, not to mention our sex lives. The cozzis are to die for and men are always entranced by belly dancers. What is more you do NOT have to be extremely large to become an excellent belly dancer.

The UK's best known belly dancer, the tiny but perfectly formed JACQUELINE CHAPMAN, RGN ONC (020 8300 76 16, www.bellydancer.org.uk) teaches at DANCEWORKS in Central London as well as South East London, Marlborough, Oxford and will perform or teach anywhere upon request. JACQUELINE also regularly visits Egypt, Turkey and Morocco and has a network of belly dancing teachers and performers all over the world. She explains more in the panel opposite.

THE HEALTH ASPECTS OF BELLY DANCING

from Jacqueline Chapman

Dance is fitness

In common with other forms of aerobic activities, oriental dancing will strengthen the lungs and heart. Many moves, especially shimmying will improve the circulation, leading to better skin conditions.

My "Mirage Method" of oriental dancing will improve total body awareness, especially of the pelvic floor muscles, beneficial to the gynaecological area. The pelvic floor muscles, when exercised, incorporate awareness of the vagina, bladder and intestines. Stress incontinence, constipation and sexual activity can be helped greatly when these exercises are practised.

The dance-form requires total concentration. It can, therefore, be therapeutic in cases of tension and depression, giving the student "time-off" regarding her problems.

Middle Eastern dancing when combined with healthy eating will aid weight reduction. Re-shaping of the waist, hips, abdominal and thigh areas will occur quite naturally. With isolation techniques taught in the "Mirage Method", breasts will become toned-up and firmer. Exercising the joints will help prevent stiffness, often found in arthritis and rheumatism.

The internal organs are massaged with movement. The glands are stimulated, leading to youthfulness, in my opinion.

If monthly misery pains are a problem, some movements stimulate abdominal activity and can help the flow during a period, alleviating pain. Total and isolated body awareness is invaluable in calming a nervous disposition, whilst allowing a strong personality to progress and experience new feelings that induce confidence. Acquiring new skills is invaluable for improving self-image.

Regular exercise and/or dancing will increase energy levels and improve stamina. The toning effect and strengthening of the pelvic floor muscles used in pregnancy and child-birth also helps to regain shape and muscle-tone after child-birth.

I teach correct posture which helps both mental and physical image. Incorrect

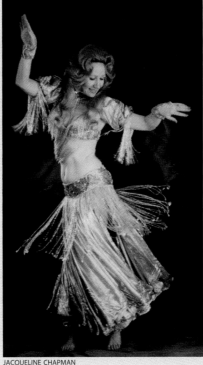

JACQUELINE CHAPMAN

posture puts pressure on the joints, in particular the spine. Correct posture allows internal organs to function properly in their natural positions.

The dance-form can be helpful in "Repetitive Strain Injury". As dancing uses all the sides of the body, it can be corrective if over-use of the body is prevalent, especially during work such as by musicians (especially violinists), painters, snooker-players, housewives, dog-grooms, and so on.

Regular weight bearing exercise increases bone mass, helping to reduce bone loss. Osteoporosis affects both women and men. Women over 35 may suffer from gradual bone loss. Thin bones fracture easily, as well as being painful and dangerous.

For an audience, watching a visual art-form can be pure escapism, allowing relaxation from everyday pressures. Developing and learning a new skill builds self-confidence. Only the individual can attend classes, discipline themselves to concentrate and learn. Therefore, respecting oneself for accepting a new goal and achiev-

ing it, is a wonderful reward. All too often low self-esteem blocks out pride and personality. Finding a hobby that can be enjoyed and even conquered can alter a person's life.

Everyone has something that pulls their heart strings – listening to opera, riding a horse – my love is dancing. Find a hobby that you can fall in love with. I feel in love with belly dancing and it has never failed me.

I can't wait to get to work whether its for performing, teaching or creating choreography. I am delightfully addicted. I am blessed with a wonderful job. I teach women to move like a dream and feel beautiful. It is unnecessary to look beautiful in order to "feel" beautiful. I believe that being fit, healthy and happy helps us to enjoy life's pleasures and cope with life's problems.

Dancers are usually fit, busy people with great legs and are rarely overweight. Belly dancing is ageless: my youngest was 5 – my oldest 90; shapeless: size 6 – 22 attend classes; sizeless: tall, short, fat, thin, wide, narrow; sexless: belly dancing is Middle Eastern folk dancing and all folk do it – men, women and children.

In my opinion, the greatest beauty secret is to be in love. For me I am in love with husband, children, home, friends and belly dancing. Love as though you have never been hurt. Dance with your heart, as though no-one is watching you.

So get belly dancing, ladies and give your partners a surprise sensual pleasure!

YOGA AND YOHM

from Heidi Meyer

Yohm is an acronym for Your Own Health Management and a new, sophisticated total well being concept that will "home deliver" a highly qualified yoga technician to any door anywhere throughout central London and soon all over Britain. (Much like a pizza only substantially better for you.)

Celebrities who have been taught yoga by YOHM teachers include:

Mariella Frostrup, Ralph Fiennes, Sadie Frost, Jade Jagger, Kate Moss, Rachel Weisz, Kylie Minogue, Danni Minogue, Madonna, Gwyneth Paltrow, Sting and Trudie Styler, Monica Belluci, Mariah Carey, Jules Oliver, Liz Hurley, Hugh Grant, Jemima Khan, Jerry Hall.

The practice of Yoga dates back over 5,000 years to the ancient dwellers of Northern India. Observing nature and searching within themselves they evolved physical postures and breathing exercises which stretched, cleansed and centred the body, cultivating states of vitality, clarity and focus.

Yoga was for many years associated with having to eat large amounts of tofu, make strict spiritual observances, and be waif enough to turn yourself into an upside down pretzel. No longer a requirement, Health Goddesses can now enjoy the benefits of civilised Yoga with Yohm. This forward thinking Yoga company brings the benefits of an ancient practice into a modern world.

Taught "one on one" in the privacy of your own home, office, hotel suite, or jet, a highly qualified Yohm Yoga technician will arrive neatly equipped with yoga mats, music, candles and chimes in tow. Beginner, intermediate, or Houdini, a blissful experience for the mind, body and soul ensues. Try a yoga party with fellow Goddesses, or escape on a luxurious Yoga and Detox minibreak.

Below are some of the wider known benefits of Yoga with Yohm. Consider it as an "essential" practice when embarking on morphing one's self into a Health Goddess.

Stress relief, Mind centering, Supple joints, Toned facial tissue, Wrinkle prevention, Energy, Vitality, Enhanced digestion, Weight loss, Migraine prevention, Freedom from back pain, Improved sleep patterns, Corrected posture, Control of menstrual pangs and pains, Recovery from ongoing fatigue, Strengthened eyesight, Relief from desk strain, Reduced birth pain, Increased recovery of pelvic floor muscles post birth, Release from pre- and post-natal depression, Improved lung capacity – relief from Asthma, Removed anxiety, Improved respiration, Better circulation, Prevention of varicose veins, Relief from depression, Release from addiction, Colon cleaning, Detoxification, Improvement of existing fitness, Prevention of Osteoporosis and Arthritis, Injury recovery and prevention, Increased longevity, Peace of mind, Bliss.

Here's what happens to you physically during a Yohm Yoga class:

Muscles including the heart, are contracted and stretched at a cellular, biochemical level. Lipids and proteins reorganise optimally in such stretching, allowing for better circulation.

Joint mobility and range of motion is increased and strength is built by the use of gravity. Muscles and joints are balanced.

Blood and calcium are brought to the bones. Working against gravity strengthens the bones. The organs of the immune system within the bones (red marrow) are boosted.

The lymph nodes are massaged, lymph is pumped throughout the body and white blood cells are distributed throughout as the lymphatic system works more efficiently. There is compression and extension to the **thymus, spleen, appendix and intestines; lungs** are stretched and flushed out by increased oxygen uptake and blood circulation. The endocrine glands are encouraged to secrete appropriate hormones and the communication between hormones and various glands and systems of the body is perfected. **Toxins and waste are eliminated** through the organs of elimination.

The nerves are stimulated by compression and extension, improving communication within the systems of the body and supplying fresh blood, oxygen and nutrients throughout.

The brain and skin are stimulated by improved circulation, oxygen intake, and by varying blood pressure.

Meditation during class creates quietness for the mind. Our relaxation revitalises the soul and you are left refreshed and glowing as a result of the experience as a whole.

The foundation of Yohm's healthy concept begins with the undertaking of regular, personable and impeccably taught yoga classes available at times that are convenient to you. You do not need to eat lentils, have matted hair or be any shape, size or age to enjoy the benefits of Yoga.

Yohm's personalised yoga concept is complemented by a range of additional and carefully thought out healthy lifestyle services designed to embrace your entire state of being. Taking into account the various principles surrounding ultimate health such as what you eat, how you grocery shop, the clutter within your home and your state of mind are all important to Yohm.

Begin living the healthy lifestyle you have always imagined. Choose from several luxurious and exciting yoga fitness and health holidays and weekends with Yohm, both in Britain and around the world. Health and Fitness Retreats for kids as hosted by Yohm and Linford Christie and Yohm Mummy and Baby Retreats for stressed and tired mummies are popular.

Yoga

YOGA is more popular than ever these days with all sorts of super fit devotees such as MADONNA having adopted it. There are lots of yoga classes available nationwide but if you live in London you simply must try HEIDI MEYER's personalised YOHM yoga experience (YOHM Limited, 33–34 Chiswell Street, London W1G 9PW, phone 0845 456 6398, www.yohm.co.uk).

Heidi explains YOHM in the panel opposite.

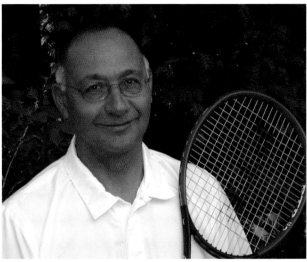

AL HILL

Tennis

TENNIS is the most fun and social sport I can think of and is also a terrific form of exercise. Playing tennis on a beautiful summer's day is extremely sensually pleasurable and whacking that little ball over the net is certainly satisfying. If you play often and hard and you do not have a two handed backhand, compensate by using your non-tennis arm more off the court as God forbid you should have one arm more developed than the other! AL HILL (07973 21 30 91, al.hill@btinternet.com), head Pro at HOLMES PLACE knows everything there is to know about tennis and told me:

"**Health** – *Tennis is mostly out doors and fresh air is great for skin, lungs and disposition. New tennis is so much faster than it used to be, so lots of running to chase balls and returning them increases lung capacity and strengthens the heart – remember the treatment for heart attack patients in America was to get them on bikes exercising.*

Another basic health rule is that expending energy creates energy and therefore makes you more energetic. And finally it is fun and you are enjoying yourself and having a laugh. All of this makes you feel better, happier and healthier.

Balance and Co-ordination – *Volleying and serving require players to hit balls that fly in the air – it takes extreme brain concentration and eye hand co-ordination and balance which always needs improving.*

Fitness – *Because tennis is faster you are now running and changing direction for longer periods during a game. A player runs forwards, backwards and sideways in quick bursts of speed. I compare this to an aerobic gym exercise with more skill required to hit a ball at the same time. Also when hitting the balls, players are using their torsos to gain more power and speed, this is building core strength in the same way as when you join a yoga and Pilates class.*"

Swimming and water sports

SWIMMING AND WATER SPORTS are also fun and sensually pleasurable ways of keeping fit, healthy and toned. Swimming is probably the best sport of all for exercising your whole body and is very safe as the water supports you. It is an excellent form of exercise if you have any injuries, particularly for back problems and there are loads of beautiful pools around nowadays.

For instance many of the HOLMES PLACE group of health and fitness clubs have swimming pools (020 7786 7300 or go to: wwww.holmesplace.com to find your nearest one). The chain has clubs throughout the UK and Europe, many with pools, tennis courts and even golf courses. My local HOLMES PLACE, FULHAM (Normand Park, Lillie Road, SW6 7ST, phone 020 7471 0450) has an excellent swimming programme presided over by former Australian Commonwealth Games gold medallist GLEN HEINDKE. The facilities at this club (the old FULHAM POOLS), including a children's pool, are also open to the public so there is no excuse not to swim regularly if you live in my neighbourhood.

Surfing is extremely energetic and water skiing and wake boarding are excellent for the legs. But scuba diving is the aqua sport which will really get you fit and make you lose weight; you do not feel as if you are exercising at all but just carrying the tank both in and out of the water will do it every time. Plus you can enjoy the sensual pleasure of being in a different dimension, "the life aquatic", the beauty of the sun on the surface of the water above you, the stunning sea life… there is nothing quite like scuba diving.

Skiing and snowboarding

SKIING AND SNOWBOARDING are the best sports for toning up the bum and thighs: you can really feel the old "thigh rubber" taking a beating as you wallop those moguls. In fact you will use all the muscles in your body, even your stomach ones, but particularly the arms, shoulders and back as well as the legs. The fresh mountain air is invigorating and will give you a wonderful appetite and the sensual pleasure of carving through the sparkling powder beneath a clear blue Alpine sky is second to none.

BRISE, the Head Ski Teacher at the ECOLE DE SKI INTERNATIONALE at Val Thorens in the Trois Vallees region of France told me *"skiing is wonderful for most people for the figure, for stamina and for the circulation. The only time when skiing is not good for you is if you have a breathing condition such as asthma".*

Health and fitness clubs

If you are pregnant or have just had a baby (or babies!) you will need to do special, more gentle exercises. You must concentrate on strengthening your thighs, buttocks and abdomen for the birth and in regaining your shape and muscle tone after your big event.

For those of you who are able to get out and about, belly dancer and former State Registered Nurse JACQUELINE CHAPMAN (020 8300 7616), who has four children herself, runs six week courses called "Belly Babies: Pre- and Post-Natal Classes with a difference" in various locations.

If you prefer to stay at home during this time of your life, there are lots of good videos available for pre and post-natal women including my very own "REGAIN YOUR FIGURE: Easy Exercises For Expectant And New Mothers" (available from Farmingham Productions, 12 Tilton Street, London, SW6 7LP, phone 020 7381 5735)

Several gyms and health clubs run pre and post-natal classes and have creches for babies and young children, including my local HOLMES PLACE, mentioned earlier. In fact HOLMES PLACES are probably the best clubs for women to join because, as well as their excellent restaurant facilities, they also offer a wide selection of both beauty treatments including waxing, manicures, pedicures and ST TROPEZ airbrush tanning and therapies including physiotherapy, acupuncture, chiropractice, homeopathy, nutritional advice, podiatry, reflexology, shiatsu and sports massages.

After all we all need a bit of pampering after exercising, not to mention a nutritious meal. HOLMES PLACE, FULHAM also has alcohol on offer but, once you get going with your sport and exercise, ladies, you should find that you will get a natural "high" and will not need to "alter your state" nearly so much! (Two units a day is plenty for a health goddess even if you are into the sensual pleasure of imbibing champagne as I must admit I am.)

Getting back to the important consideration of finding a good health and fitness club, I like the holistic approach at the HOLMES PLACES. You are given a proper induction: a "starter programme". There are loads of different classes (even Salsa dancing) and personal trainers and you can work out in a women's only gym if your hair and make-up are not up to joining the unisex one or you are a new recruit and want a bit of privacy. The clubs call themselves "destination places" where you can enjoy yourself with all the family, plus they offer children's and young people's memberships for the young girls amongst you.

I talked to DAVID THOMAS, the manager of HOLMES PLACE/FULHAM, a former England International squash player and ALUN THOMAS (no relation!) the assistant manager and a fitness and nutritional expert and they exploded a few myths for me.

"Some fitness and nutrition myths

In general 60% of weight loss (if you are trying to lose weight) is effected by nutrition not exercise but of course exercise is very good for you. It is a fallacy that good exercising builds up too much muscle in women. Females have hardly any testosterone in their bodies so they do not bulk up in the same way as men.

However one in three women in this country are at risk of getting osteoporosis and weight bearing exercise, including weight training, will help to significantly decrease the risk of getting it in later life.

Nutrition is all important. Organic food is significantly better than ordinary food. At the moment it may be more expensive but it is becoming cheaper all the time due to the competition in this area of food production. If you eat organically, or at least healthily, you should not need to take any vitamins or other food supplements unless you are a strict Vegan, an elite athlete or have some sort of deficiency.

All weight loss diets are cleverly marketed but you must find out which is best for you: for instance the ATKINS diet would work well if you can tolerate a lot of protein, which not everybody can.

In general people do not drink enough water, although you need to find out how much is right for you. The risks of over drinking are much less than those of dehydration. However there is a difference between ordinary water and 'metabolic water' which is found in the foods we eat. We need to eat plenty of fruit and vegetables which contain this metabolic water.

Of course the more you drink the more you will need to go to the toilet, although this is good for flushing out toxins in your diet. However when PAULA RADCLIFFE famously had to take a 'loo stop' at around the twenty mile mark in the LONDON MARATHON 2005 it was probably because she had drunk too much water before the race. When you are doing that sort of endurance test or indeed any exercise involving long exertion, such as playing tennis for two hours, you should drink an 'isotonic' energy drink, which contains sugar, salt and glucose which gets absorbed quickly into your system, instead of loads of water. The new LUCOZADE is a good isotonic drink, for instance.

In general, however, it is fine to drink water throughout your exercise and do not forget the basic rules of not eating a big meal within two hours of exercising (although you can have a banana or energy bar for instant energy just before) and eating within two hours (preferably less) afterwards to replenish your energy levels. You should do this even if you are trying to lose weight; exercising allows you to eat more (as long as you eat the right foods and not too much alcohol) without feeling guilty. Really it is a lifestyle choice: there is no point going to the gym if you do not eat properly. Also there is no point taking out a membership of a health club if you do not keep it up. You must be disciplined."

Well said, guys! Working out is a discipline and whoever said "exercise is for life" was correct because you just do not feel or look so good if you give it up.

Natural secrets

GEORGINA BRUNI, my Editor-in-Chief at HOT GOSSIP UK gave me the great little recipe at the left for a healthy citrus drink which will get you up and at 'em and ready for your exercise routine in the morning (use honey not sugar if you can – it tastes just as good):

MORNING ENERGY BOOST

from Georgina Bruni

GEORGINA BRUNI

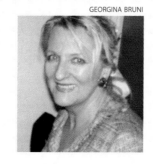

1 large orange.

1 lemon

1 grapefruit

1 Tbsp sugar or honey to taste

6 ice cubes

Glass of water

Some rind

Overleaf are some great home based facial and body exercises and lifestyle tips from one of my esteemed publishers, TATIANA VON SAXE, a fully fledged health goddess who just adores sensual pleasures:

At HOT GOSSIP UK I get a huge post bag from Asian ladies who say their diet and lifestyle makes them put on weight as they get older. This does not have to be so: here is a report from popular Asian TV star RANI SINGH whom we all know and love from "EASTENDERS", etc. (Jaffrey Kent representation, phone 01753 785 162; Curtis Brown representation, phone 020 7393 4400) and who always looks fantastic:

RANI SINGH

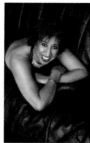

©JOHN DAWSON

"While Asian women are often gifted with skins which do not show their age, and are sometimes considered to be amongst the world's most beautiful women (ref. consistent number of top three finalists for Miss World and Miss Universe over the years), being a (South) Asian woman is also like being an Exocet missile genetically designed to self-destruct.

Not only are depression and the suicide rates highest amongst the UK Asian female population compared to any other community, the British Heart Foundation has found that Asian women are 51 per cent more likely to die from coronary heart disease than the rest of the UK population.

The problem is related to high levels of cholesterol and a lack of exercise. This even applies to second generation (South) Asians and the trend is continuing. Asian culture and home life are meal-orientated; (South) Asians for instance love an excuse to party and there are festivals for almost every day of the year! Personally I have the added stress of needing to look my best whenever I am on show, particularly when there are cameras around.

Once we pass our early twenties it is important that we start to take notice of what we are doing to our bodies. Counselling and personal training, regular exercise and diet watch are not natural features of Asian lives. I cope with the pressures of my lifestyle by making sure to have all of them in mine. Doing multiple retakes on a big film set or recording five TV programmes back to back in half a day requires stamina and concentration.

Exercise can take many forms. I like the social aspect of group exercise and played for my school teams at Haberdashers Aske's School in Elstree where sport was big. Classical Indian dance training during my Performance Arts Degree also kept

THE NATURAL WAY

from Tatiana von Saxe

If you have been lucky and learned at an early age, both at home and at school, about real values then you have the perfect foundation to become a Health Goddess.

Respect, in my view is one of the secrets for everything. Your life will flourish with an enduring quality that will make the difference between just existing and fulfilment. It will improve your relationship with everybody.

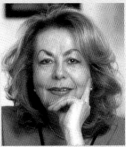

TATIANA VON SAXE

Everything in moderation is the other secret. So even if you indulge from time to time if done in moderation it will not create permanent damage. Damage can also occur by having too much of a good thing. Not everyone needs 3 litres of water a day – listen to your metabolism. Not everyone needs hours in the gym – do what comes naturally to you.

DEVOTE 15 MINUTES PER DAY TO YOURSELF AND DO THE FOLLOWING:

Five minutes of facial exercises:

1 Sprinkle water on your face and close your eyes.
Close your mouth and force your lips forward as if throwing a kiss to someone: hold that position for 20 seconds.
Open your eyes as if you are very surprised. Open your mouth wide as if you are yawning. Hold for 20 seconds.
Repeat two more times, alternating.
Total: two minutes

2 Position your front teeth in front of your lower ones with your mouth shut. Hold to a count of four. Change and position your lower teeth in front of your upper ones. Hold to a count of four. Repeat to a total count of 36.
Then hold to a count of two and repeat ten times.
Total: one minute

3 Sprinkle some water on your face.
Close your mouth and force your lips tightly closed. Puff out your cheeks as much as you can. Slap your face for two minutes.
Total: two minutes

4 Have a glass of something you love: my favourite is the detox drink I make and always keep ready for use *(Recipe below)*.

Five minutes of relaxation:

Close your eyes and sit on your most comfortable chair/sofa/bed in your most favourite place of your flat/house. Think of beautiful things. Transport yourself to wherever you want to be. Visualise yourself in whichever way you would like to be. Indulge in your comfort zone.
Total: five minutes

Five minutes of body exercise:

Two minutes bust and arms: position the palms of your hands together (vertically, finger tips towards ceiling) in front of your chest and press hard together to a count of three and release. Repeat for one minute.
Cross your arms in front of your chest – wrap both hands around the opposite wrist. Press in and out as hard as you can to a count of ten. Rest. Repeat four times

One minute back: The pelvic tilt – lie on the floor with your arms at your sides, feet flat on the floor and your legs bent. Gently press the back of your waist against the floor and tilt your pelvis forward by tightening the abdominal and buttock muscles. Hold for six seconds. Relax for two seconds. Repeat six times.

One minute stomach: Sitting or standing up: Breath in and force your stomach muscles inwards while contracting your buttocks. Hold to a count of ten. Exhale. Repeat five times.

One minute legs: Go up and down the stairs for 60 seconds – try using the stairs instead of lifts wherever you go.

GOOD HEALTH BROTH (DETOX DRINK)

INGREDIENTS

As many vegetables as you like. Do not peel them or remove stalks/leaves but wash them thoroughly. You can also use vegetable peelings from vegetables you will be using for a meal. The best: potatoes (dark skin preferably), onions, asparagus (not necessarily the tips which can be used as a vegetable), white radish, carrots, celery, pea pods, corn on the cob (with kernels), parsnips, turnips, broccoli stalks (not the flowers which can be used as a vegetable), 3 cloves of garlic (unpeeled).

METHOD

Place ingredients in an earthenware pot (never use metal cooking utensils) and cover with three parts water. Boil until mixture is reduced by half. Put mixture through a sieve and keep the broth. Throw the vegetables away except the potatoes that can be peeled and used for mashing.

Make it a habit to:

- Eat only fresh produce (do not use microwaves)
- Have delicious vegetables prepared in the fridge for nibbling.
- Have a jug of the Good Health broth to drink hot or cold.

me flexible, but after that working in mainstream television and film didn't give me a daily structure for health and exercise (indeed it's hard to do body maintenance with location food, tight deadlines and all night sessions in studios and newsrooms) so I work hard at staying healthy and finding what works for me.

Sportsmen and women make great Personal Trainers and generally sport-orientated countries like South Africa, the USA and Australia produce some excellent ones.

My own needs arise from the typically hectic actress/presenter lifestyle with obligatory awards dinners with hard-to-resist desserts and chocolates with the coffee. My all-time favourite Trainer is South African Dave Arton-Powell. Athletes have to lead disciplined lives, and Arton-Powell himself was a competitive body-builder, triathlete and swimmer. He's taught me I don't need to spend hours in the gym or go on a starvation diet. The idea is to train intensively past my comfort zone, particularly with cardio work, to keep my heart rate up and to take short rests not long ones.

I need a simple programme and have limited time to spend in the gym so Dave designed one for me with just a few weights machines dividing two sessions of cardio work – I can do it all in under an hour.

He's also taught me the importance of careful diet (but allows me a cheat day once a week). I eat four or five meals a day to help raise my metabolism and stop energy dips.

Of course the golden rule of drinking around two litres of water per day is important but Dave points out that getting thirsty and hungry are signs of stomach starvation so I try to keep myself topped up all the time with regular drinks and food. He makes sure I stay in good health especially during and after heavy filming schedules.

And of course regular exercise increases the amount of seratonin (the feel good chemical) levels in the brain which encourage us to do more exercise and improve. Very pertinent for all (South) Asians, not just those of us in showbiz!

Note: Personal Trainer Dave Arton-Powell can be contacted at: dartonpowell@hotmail.co.uk"

Pilates

You should always protect your back when you are exercising or playing sport. The spine is the centre of the body and is actually quite delicate. If you have a weak back you should use the back machine at your local gym to build up the muscles surrounding your spine and be careful to keep your back curled when doing your abdominal exercises.

PILATES is a popular exercise system which is particularly beneficial for back problems. You can find PILATES classes at various clubs nowadays including at the HOLMES PLACES. You should also use a chair that supports your back properly when slaving over your hot computer, etc. and do go straight to the osteopath or a chiropractor if you have any sort of back pain whatsoever.

Here is a report from chiropractor IDA NORGAARD DC, MSc, SCC (33 Thurloe Place, London SW7 2HQ, phone 020 7581 5671, www.fix-a-spine.co.uk):

BACK PAIN
from Ida Norgaard, Chiropractor

What general factors contribute to back pain?

The neck and back function to provide stability, strength, endurance, flexibility, co-ordination and balance. Dysfunction may involve disturbances to any of these functions as well as more local problems in joints, muscles, ligaments and tendons. Most back or neck pain can be attributed to this dysfunction, which simply means that joints and muscles, as well as the nervous system itself, are not performing their job as efficiently as they could.

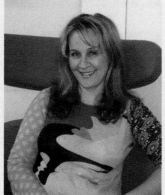

IDA NORGAARD

Joint dysfunction

This occurs when one or more of the joints in the spine, or in a leg, loses its resilience or ability to absorb shock. It can also happen when joints are overloaded by such things as poor posture and lose their centred alignment. When joint dysfunction develops, the normal range or pattern of movement is affected and the joint may become inflamed. Once inflamed, pain receptors in the joint itself become sensitised – as a result, even the slightest movement can make the nerves fire spontaneously, causing pain in the joint. Also, because the joint contains many different nerve receptors, dysfunction can send abnormal signals to the central nervous system, causing muscle imbalance around the joint.

Muscle imbalance

Once a pain cycle has been established, deconditioning –in the form of muscle spasms, joint stiffness and muscle weakness – is the inevitable result. Some muscles respond to joint dysfunction by becoming tense and overactive, while others respond by becoming limp and under active. In both cases the affected muscles can exacerbate pain and dysfunction.

Faulty movement patterns, poor posture and overload

When you have poor posture, the body overloads the joints and muscles that work together to produce specific movements and, as a result, they no longer cooperate to ensure smooth and painless action – this is how a faulty movement pattern is created. This can cause muscles and joints to weaken. While these faults in movement patterns can directly involve the back, they can also come from or lead to dysfunction in other areas of the body, such as the hip, knee or foot. Regardless of where they originate, faulty movements always lead to functional limitation and an inability to perform everyday tasks without pain or discomfort.

Disc problems

Joint and muscle dysfunction and the faulty movement patterns that follow put strain on the discs that lie between each vertebra. If a disc herniates or protrudes backwards, an inflammatory reaction occurs which may also affect a nerve. Pain in the back may then be "referred" to a buttock, leg or the foot; if it is severe, it may even cause neurological symptoms such as numbness and tingling. It may eventually lead to muscle wasting.

How does the Chiropractor know what is causing my back pain?

Chiropractors are trained to identify significant joint and muscle dysfunction, faulty movement patterns and disc problems, as well as

other disorders that may be affecting your well-being. A key element in treating pain is the successful diagnosis and subsequent treatment programme for the overloaded tissues.

Medical history

Before beginning treatment, your chiropractor may ask you to fill in a questionnaire relating to your back pain as well as ask you in depth questions about your back pain and general health. Using this detailed information, the chiropractor can rule out any potentially serious contributing factors and direct the examination to the real issues that may be causing your pain.

Physical examination

Your chiropractor will observe your posture and movement patterns and examine your muscles and joints as well as performing a neurological examination and general physical tests such as blood pressure etc. Palpation is the chiropractor's means of establishing how well joints and muscles are functioning by demonstrating resistance, tension, friction and tightness. Motion palpation is used to establish joint movement restrictions.

Testing

Occasionally, it is necessary to obtain advanced testing such as X-Rays, CT scans, MRI scans or blood tests to investigate the problem further and rule out any serious underlying causes.

In most cases, after this testing routine is complete, a diagnosis can be established. If the problem is determined to be treatable, an individualised treatment strategy will be formulated and discussed with you in detail, so you fully understand the options available to you.

What will my treatment consist of?

Most back or neck pain is not serious and will respond to straightforward treatment. Your chiropractor can accurately diagnose and effectively treat most types of back pain in their office. Your treatment strategy will be uniquely designed to your particular needs and directed at the primary dysfunctions that were detected during your examination.

The most common treatments are:

Spinal manipulation

Manipulation is a general term used to describe a variety of techniques. Chiropractors use the term "adjustment" to describe a procedure that is used to normalise joint function. This consists of gently moving the affected joint and may also involve the application of a short, quick push or pull in the direction of the restriction. In contrast, mobilisation is the use of slow repetitive stretching movements to release the restricted joint or muscles.

Muscle relaxation/stimulation

Relaxation of the muscles consists of gentle stretches to relax the affected muscle. Repeated contractions of a weak muscle will help to reactivate and strengthen it and the application of gentle pressure to trigger points will help relieve the pain associated with these.

Rehabilitative exercises

Many chiropractors now advise a programme of exercises, designed to help achieve quick but lasting pain relief. A programme of exercises is prescribed to "re-program" movement patterns so they will become subconscious. The goal is to focus the exercise on specific muscles while using the "deep" muscles that control and guide movement.

Respiration

Improving your respiratory function is no less important than improving the strength of the muscles in your back and your posture or joint function. Breathing in the upper part of your chest is one of the most frequent perpetuating factors in repetitive strain to both the neck and low back which subsequently causes headaches, neck pain and backaches.

Stabilisation/sensorimotor training

These are exercises that are designed to train your nervous system to co-ordinate and control routine, everyday movement patterns. They are also designed to improve the ability of the muscles supporting your spine to maintain their stability which is crucial for all other movements.

Workplace (ergonomic) and lifestyle advice

Millions of people suffer from neck or back pain for which they can't find a specific cause. Often this is due to "repetitive strain" from occupational overuse. The human body was not designed to stay in one constrained position for prolonged periods of time. It requires motion and activity to maintain circulation and keep muscles relaxed. The pain may start suddenly or gradually but the problem was inevitably developing for months, years or even decades before the onset of pain.

Education

Education is an essential part of the treatment and prevention of back pain. Many chiropractors offer regular back-care classes covering anatomy, posture, body mechanics and exercise programmes as well as "first aid" – should an injury happen again.

Posture

The importance of posture is often forgotten. You cannot be truly healthy if you do not hold yourself correctly and you will never look like a goddess if you slump or have round shoulders! Exercise (especially dancing) will help you to attain and maintain correct posture so that you will feel and look better and clothes always hang better on a nice straight body.

PILATES and THE ALEXANDER TECHNIQUE, both of which are available in lots of different clubs, will help your posture considerably. Alternatively walk around with a book on your head, a method which some "young ladies' academies" still employ for dealing with their slouching "WAYNETTAs"! You will soon be walking with a truly goddess like glide. Below is what IDA has to say on the subject of posture:

POSTURE

from Ida Norgaard, Chiropractor

Usually many of us find ourselves more slouched forward than we would like to be for too much of the time and we catch ourselves doing it more often and for longer. It may start sitting in the office or in front of the television or the computer but all of a sudden it is a constant fixture and very difficult to change.

While poor posture ruins the look of even the most beautiful dress and generally makes it impossible to look elegant, it also prevents using our stomach and back muscles properly. When slouching, we change the way we breathe from the diaphragm to the upper chest. Not using the diaphragm stops the abdominal muscles responding correctly and we pull the upper part of the abdomen under the ribcage so that the ribs in front start to poke out and a small belly forms that will not respond even to a million crunches.

As we breathe with the upper chest, we develop tension in the neck muscles and start to stick the chin forward. This can and will eventually be more than just an unpleasant cosmetic issue. It is frequently the cause of headache, neck pain, a stiff shoulder, numbness or tingling in an arm, pain between the shoulder blades, difficulty in breathing properly and even lower back pain.

Posture ranks high on the list when you are talking about good health, fitness and looking and feeling good. Good posture is a way of doing things with more energy and less strain, stress and fatigue. Without good posture you cannot really be physically fit and look good. The human body is designed for movement. Keeping in one position for an extended period of time increases stiffness and tension. As a result sitting is a common cause of lower back and neck pain.

When we think of activities that are "bad" for the back, strenuous things such as lifting, bending and certain sports usually come to mind. However a prolonged static posture such as sitting is also extremely bad for the back.

For most us, life involves a computer either at home or at work. Just about everybody uses one. Sitting slouched or slumped forward increases disc pressure and exhausts muscles and ligaments in your neck, shoulder and back – even for as short a time as 15–20 minutes.

A lifetime of poor posture can start a progression of symptoms, including muscle tiredness with your muscles having to work hard to hold you up. You change the load on joints, tightening muscles further and using the joints in an inefficient way, predisposing yourself to headache, neck pain, stiff shoulders, lower back pain and osteoporosis in later years, thus increasing the likelihood of compression fractures in the spine.

What does good posture look like?

Perfect posture is individual. Everybody's body is different but as a test you should be able to stand with the back of your head, shoulder blades, buttocks and heels against the wall without lifting the chest, arching the back or moving the neck from the wall.

How to practise good posture?

Use the wall as your reference. Stand with your heels and buttocks against the wall, keeping the weight on both the heel and the front of your foot where the big toe meets the foot. Keep your feet hip width apart and gently squeeze the thighs towards each other whilst "rolling" them outwards from the tops of the legs at the same time (as if you were trying to turn the legs outwards but the squeezing "together" of the thighs prevents you).

Now take a deep breath in, then release the breath and pull down the shoulder blades (towards the back pocket, not together) and flatten the back against the wall and slide your head back. (It may help if you have your palms facing forward and reach downward with the arms and add a little force to breathing out.)

Once you master this against the wall, practise while waiting for the bus or tube or for the kettle to boil. Carry your shopping home in this posture. It will wake up the muscles in the back of your arms and across the shoulder blades as well as the deep muscles in the abdomen and lower back.

Posture breaks when sitting:
take frequent breaks and get up and move around.

Sit on the edge of your chair, feet and knees hip width apart. As you prepare yourself, gently squeeze thighs together while rolling the knees outward without actually moving the legs. Slide your chin backwards, neither looking down or up. Take a deep breath in.

Keep the shoulder blades pulled down towards the back pockets, palms facing forwards and arms just coming in front of

the hips. As you breathe out, use a little force and concentrate on sliding the chin back and rolling the arms/palms out and away from you.

Breathing out while doing this little postural exercise stops you from just lifting the chest and arching the lower back and helps to straighten the spine.

Repeat as often as you can when sitting or at least once an hour.

Feldenkrais method – pains and injuries

Talking about bad backs and posture leads me to the world famous FELDENKRAIS METHOD, a remarkable discipline which can help with all sorts of pain and injuries from repetitive strain injuries (RSI) to accident trauma. Here senior FELDENKRAIS practitioner ORNA DALE-ELIASHIV (07747 185318, orna59@yahoo.com) tells us all about FELDENKRAIS below and on the following pages.

FELDENKRAIS
from Orna Dale-Eliashiv

Habits, posture, and freedom

The Feldenkrais Method is one of the most beneficial, effective and friendly disciplines ever devised. The method creates remarkable improvements in the motor system with an incredible economy of means. It uses awareness to reach out to movement and movement to reach out to awareness. Both improve together while improving each other and with them is enhanced the general well-being and capacity for comfort and pleasure.

The depth and power of the method emanate from western and eastern scientific knowledge and inspiration. It was invented by Dr Moshe Feldenkrais, master of martial arts, physicist and a man of very original thought; a brilliant practitioner as well as a most inspirational and intuitive teacher.

Who is the method most beneficial for?

The method addresses both women and men who want to enjoy a healthy and vital life and particularly want to improve the following: ease and range of movement, flexibility, agility, posture, balance, co-ordination, optimism and self-image.

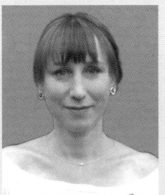

ORNA DALE-ELIASHIV

The method also helps in relieving back/knee/neck and joint pains, muscular tension that comes from routine work, repetitive strain injuries and skeletal problems like slipped disc and scoliosis (mis-alignment of the spine). It helps to improve circulation, breathing and the metabolism. It also helps to prevent injuries and aids recuperation. In the emotional dimension: it helps low concentration, impatience, stress and depressed mood. In the care of children: the method assists children in their development, helping them

become aware of their body and guiding them in their ability to control it. Children with developmental problems such as dyslexia, problems with spatial awareness and balance, or developmental problems with basic functions such as crawling, sitting, standing or walking could be helped by the method and could reach improvement and personal achievement in the physical, emotional and mental areas.

Lastly, there are special areas: palliative treatment of the symptoms of MS, brain damage and accident trauma.

The power of the Feldenkrais Method is that it pushes out the limits of ability in an indirect and comfortable way. It's not interested in effort, stress or pain, but in ease and pleasure. Its concern is that your movement and functioning will hit the bulls eye through the principle of "minimum effort, maximum efficiency". Feldenkrais says "…what you know how to do well is not hard to do; or alternatively, what's hard to do is not being done well". On top of this you have got to add: what's not done well will soon lead to pain, and the more effort you make, the sooner the pain comes.

A person taking Feldenkrais lessons becomes familiar with a new and efficient way of moving. This results in a very noticeable gain in movement ability, reduction of pain and tension and a deep influence on the general sensation of well-being. Feldenkrais compared this "tuning" of the body to the tuning of a piano, commenting that even the best musician can't make a good sound on an out-of-tune instrument.

As a master of martial arts, Feldenkrais understood that the ultimate test of movement is efficiency. This principle can be seen working for a soldier defending against superior forces, or for an actor who can hypnotise us from the minute he steps on the stage (including the stage of life), as well as for each person who wants to get through a hard day and not pay for it with a bad back. In all of these cases there is bodily freedom and they look to us effortless and naturally graceful. I can assure you that these qualities exist inside all of us – they're just waiting for the right approach to bring them out.

None of us had to go to school to learn to sit, to turn, to walk, or to jump. We learned all these tricks subconsciously in an effortless and natural way. It's like a mother tongue which is never forgotten. As children we used our bodies to try out all sorts of different moves that we discovered for ourselves. We were a great joy but also a bit of a strain on our loving and exhausted parents: our sheer inventiveness in our physical activity had no limits, and had our parents run off their feet by the end of the day. We were all able to take on such a huge learning curve because of the innate human capacity to change and to develop.

As we grow into adults we learn to adapt ourselves to the demands of life; we restrict our range of movements to what seems suitable. And so we end up with habits of behaviour, peculiar to us as our handwriting, which we are not aware of any more. Habits can be very dominant in our lives; they supply security, flow and identity. You can't live without them but sometimes you can't live with them! Some of our habits bring with them a hidden disorganization that spoils the natural flow and elegance of movement and creates a limitation in our ability. With time they lead to pain and injuries, yet we don't know the cause. The nature of habits is that we repeat them constantly. The strange thing is that even in pain, the body's system hangs on to what it's used to, although this may actually be the reason for the pain. Why does it do it? The familiar feels comfortable and reliable, but perhaps also we don't know differently. In other words, as adults, we forgot. Bit by bit, the body forgets, gives up on trying, and eventually these little bits become a lot. Time takes its toll. So what should we do about it?

Feldenkrais Method makes very good use of the innate human capacity to change and develop which babies and children take advantage of. As we gathered habits once, we can now choose new ones. Using a series of gentle motions the Feldenkrais Method will bring back to our bodies a range of movements that were lost over time; and with them will bring back the natural grace and lightness that we all want to feel.

The student of the method gets introduced to efficient ways of movement that he wasn't able to think about for himself. He learns to notice the small details of movements that were normally hidden from his consciousness and this new awareness helps him to avoid being imprecise in his actions; both in the way he moves and the way he synergises his actions into the general pattern. While improving and refining the movement we learn to deepen the observation and the awareness and to organise ourselves in a more efficient way. The big advantage is that the system learns to tune itself; to find good solutions by its own means; to improvise and become comfortable to adjustment – so comfortable that you can trust it no less than you trust your habit. The internal freedom gets enhanced, which allows the principle of the natural creativity (which we all have) to work. I don't know of any freedom, joy or confidence better than that.

When you sit on a chair, you not only drop onto the chair, but each vertebra drops into a specific place relative to its neighbours; and so does every other bone – the thigh bone, the shin bone and even the skull. Each point in your body travels through a specific path when you change your physical position and each spot moves in concert with all the other parts of your body (face it: you don't fall apart!).

Feldenkrais asks: did each bone go through the ideal path on the way to the chair; did all the parts of the body make the best co-ordination between themselves; was there enough freedom in each joint to do the small job (or the big job, it depends on which joint and the kind of movement) that was their function. Ask yourself: did you stop breathing for a second? Did your body manage to obey your intention? More than that, did it manage to respond to your intention gracefully and easily? All of these questions can be asked about each function; about anything you want to do. In a nutshell, Feldenkrais Method is interested in the dynamic of the action, and in its quality.

An ideal posture is very rare; so rare that we can say it doesn't exist, but whether you are a dancer or your physical scope is limited, Feldenkrais Method can take you forward step by step.

When we know about the efficient ways to move from position to position, we become the master of our movements, our intentions, our bodies, and our functioning. We become a free person. We recognise the efficient way to move from position to position using our sixth sense – the kinaesthetic sense. This is our most intuitive sense, responding to our internal sensations. We want to sharpen it like a painter sharpens his sense of seeing.

Now for some details of the actual practice of Feldenkrais. The method uses two techniques; one of them is One-to-One sessions, and the other is Group lessons. First, the individual lesson, which we call Functional Integration, or F.I. In the individual lesson the student is lying on a couch or sometimes sitting on a chair. It's built around the specific needs of the student and produces quick results. The teacher uses an expert system of touching and manipulation learnt from hundreds of hours of study of the delicate details of movement; this eases tension in the muscles, and can also ease tension in the student's feelings and emotions. It's suitable for people who need urgent relief from pain; for children and babies; for people with special problems that prevent them from joining group lessons; or – to people who just love the relaxed and comfortable feeling after the lesson.

Secondly, the group lesson, known as awareness through movement, or ATM.

In the group lessons the students make movements for themselves under the verbal direction of the teacher. Group lessons are usually taken lying down. In this way the muscles can stop fighting gravity and the students are better able to develop an awareness of their sensations, their bodies and the way they are using them. Each lesson explores a specific movement theme, made of different variations of motions that may not seem related to the desired purpose, but each variation contains important elements of the end result. At the end of the lesson, all the elements spontaneously synergise into efficient, easy and confident movement. The process is gradual and pleasant; it is not supposed to be an exercise class!

The Feldenkrais Method has been around since the early 1950s. Since then it has grown into a world-wide community of many thousands of teachers and students, and has taken its rightful place in the lexicon of modern complementary medicine.

Foot care

Whatever sort of sport or exercise you are into, you will be working on your feet so do not forget about foot health. Always buy or hire the right sort of shoes for your particular sport, particularly if we are talking tennis or skiing. Plus you must take care of your feet and nails: regular chiropody sessions and pedicures are advisable to keep your feet healthy and good looking.

VICTORIA WILSON, MInstChPLCh of BEAUCHAMP FOOT & BODY CARE (41 Beauchamp Place, London SW3 1NX, phone 020 7225 0794), has some excellent advice:

FOOT CARE

from Victoria Wilson, Chiropodist

I think the most common saying we chiropodists hear from women about feet is "If your feet hurt, it shows on your face".

Therefore foot care should be at least as important as a good facial; feet are our most neglected body part. Most women spend considerable amounts of money on face creams and body products but feet seem to be the area we spend the least time and money on.

A bit of daily maintenance and some regular professional tender loving care every 6–8 weeks will keep your feet in fabulous condition.

Chiropody is more than just removing the odd corn – it's about keeping your feet comfortable, beautiful and providing all those little bits you always wished they did in a pedicure.

Daily routine

1 **Soak your feet** – if you don't have time to sit with your feet in a bowl, make sure you put the plug in while you have a shower.
2 **Moisturise** – cream your feet with a urea based product which is ideal for replenishing lost moisture. Urea is produced naturally by our bodies to moisturise our skin, so it is easily absorbed and will not leave your feet too greasy. You can get these products from chemists or chiropodists.
3 **Foot powder** – acts as a dry lubricant to help prevent friction and pressure from footwear during the day.

Twice weekly

Either apply a foot exfoliator or use a foot file in the bath.

A few **first aid tips** for whenever necessary

Cracked heels – apply Friars Balsam to clean cracks with a cotton bud.

Summer hot feet – Witch Hazel gel to cool. Foot powder in shoes to stop burning soles.

Tea Tree Oil – good for all minor infections and abrasions, including "Athlete's Foot".

For all of my secrets, you will have to come and visit me in person!

Smell 8

ARE YOU FRAGRANT?

Smelling a flower in bloom or indeed any beautiful fragrance is a delightfully sensual pleasure. Smell is also what first attracts animals to each other. Does *he* smell right? (Your boyfriend, not your pet!) In any case you must ensure that *you* smell divine, like a goddess, at all times and that everything around you is equally fragrant: your hair, your clothes, your home, your car… Perfume, scented candles, luxurious bath products must all become part of your aura as a fragrant health goddess.

Smell is so evocative and will remind you of various times in your life; your perfume should remind *him* of *you*. How to choose the fragrance or fragrances that are right for you and your skin? (Remember that, like men, there will always be more than one scent that you can live with forever.) Here is a run down on some of the most feminine and goddess like perfumes (you may prefer to call them "scents" if you are truly posh) from the top fragrance houses.

Describing the importance of fragrance, ROSA GRASSO (ELIZABETH ARDEN, 29 Davies Street, Mayfair, London W1K 4LW, phone 0870 444 1525, www.reddoorsalons.com) told me: *"Fragrant hair, attractively styled, is vital in creating the 'image' a woman wants for herself. Not unlike the feather-ruffling peacock, tossing one's hair attracts attention."*

Products

If you are a teen or pre-teen (I do not recommend the wearing of perfume by very young girls) or in your twenties you can get away with sweet young fragrances like CHANEL's "Coco Mademoiselle", LANCÔME's "Miracle So Magic", DIOR's "Diorissimo" or J-LO's "Glow". Sporty young girls will probably prefer a fresher fragrance such as CALVIN KLEIN's "ck one", REVLON's "Charlie" or CLARINS' "Eau Dynamisante". Pure perfume is not cheap for young budgets so always go for Eau de Toilette sprays; if you do not get what you want for Christmas or birthdays have a wander round BOOTS where you will find lots of cheaper brands.

More mature ladies can wear very sophisticated and sexy scents like YSL's "Rive Gauche", DIOR's "Opium", ROCHAS' "Femme", THIERRY MUGLER's aptly named "Angel", VIVIENNE WESTWOOD's "Anglomania" or VERSACE's "Woman". As you get older your skin changes and your favourite perfumes will start to smell different on you. At this stage I suggest you revert to more classic fragrances such as BULGARI's "Woman", HERMÈS' "Calèche", DIOR's "Miss Dior" (which is actually quite grown up in spite of its name), CHANEL's "No 19" and BALENCIAGA's "Bal Á Versailles".

Lovers of sweet floral scents will adore YSL's "Paris", LAGERFELD's "Chloe", GUERLAIN's "Chamade", CHANEL's "Chance" and PATOU's "Joy". Or, if money is an object, you can pick up some beautiful "Tea Rose" scents in the markets. Ladies who prefer a "green" smell should go for ESTÉE LAUDER's "Alliage" or GIORGIO OF BEVERLY HILLS' "Giorgio", one of the most popular perfumes in the world which is now sadly harder to find in the UK but you can always pick it up when you travel abroad.

New or indecisive perfume wearers should choose something "safe" that smells good on every skin, for instance

DIOR's current best-seller, "J'Adore", CHANEL's "No.5" or LANCÔME's recent but classic "Attraction". ELIZABETH ARDEN's fragrance, "Provocative Woman" is also a good all rounder which smells nice on all sorts of different skins. But if you want to smell different from all your sisters two unusual and truly memorable scents have actually been created by male designers: MICHAEL KORS' "Michael" and JOSEPH's "Joseph". Another unusual and aptly named perfume which attracts gents to ladies like bees to a honey pot is VIVIENNE WESTWOOD's very grown up "Boudoir".

The longest lasting scents seem to be the ESTÉE LAUDER ones (that "grande dame" of American fragrance knew a thing or two) and people will stop you in the street to ask what perfume you are wearing if it is her "Estée". LAUDER's "Beyond Paradise" is a modern favourite for all ages and skin types and their best seller "Beautiful" has great goddess appeal for obvious reasons.

For those of us who prefer a more ambiguous smell I suggest GUERLAIN's "Habit Rouge" which is actually a men's fragrance but smells equally fabulous on some ladies.

It is a sad fact of life that most perfumes today are not made from flowers but from more than 4,000 synthetic chemicals. If you are allergic to perfume or just want to play it safe and healthy try ECCO BELLA's "100% Natural Eau de Parfum" collection. ECCO BELLA is a new company whose name means, literally, "here, beautiful!" The ECCO BELLA fragrances are a complex blend of essential oils from flowers, fruits, herbs and spices and they smell delightfully sophisticated. Their "Bourbon Vanilla" is a true sensual pleasure and "Ambrosia" is definitely nectar for all of us goddesses! The ECCO BELLA collection is available from LEMONBURST at 01273 558 112, www.lemonburst.net

The fragrance market is a huge and confusing one so I suggest you always "try before you buy" and have fun testing scent in stores or pharmacies (or ask mail order companies if they have any mini samples to send you). Do not try more than four perfumes at any one time

and leave the scent on your skin for at least ten minutes until it changes with your individual chemistry. Never buy a perfume that smells great on someone else without trying it yourself.

If you want to be truly fragrant, your sweet smelling regime should not end with perfume and body lotions. Some make-up and skin care products smell and taste wonderful so choose those if they suit your skin. For instance most of the LANCÔME and LAUDER skin care products smell very feminine whilst the CLINIQUE range smells young and fresh. One excellent skin care product which smells unusually divine is French manufacturer GARRAUD's Hydro 24 Hour Cream which you can also buy in the US. Two other manufacturers whose products smell particularly delightful and whose ranges I will discuss in Chapter 11 are PURELOGICOL and DR DENESE. On the make-up front, most lip glosses have wonderful taste and smell appeal nowadays but the sweetest smellers are DIOR's "Diorkiss" Luscious Lip-Plumping Gloss which plumps your mouth up at the same time, LANCÔME's "Juicy Tubes" Ultra Shiny Lip Gloss and BOOTS' "Natural Collection" Lip Lickers.

Most of us like to use convenient aerosol air fresheners nowadays but they can actually make babies and their mothers ill. In fact a recent study showed that frequent use of air fresheners and aerosols during pregnancy and early childhood was associated with higher levels of diarrhoea and earache in infants as well as headaches and depression in mothers. So do not take any chances, mums: use a natural non aerosol freshener like ECCO MIST which is made from essential oils, emulsifier and water only and is available in various delightful fragrances (ring 01273 558112 for stockists).

For those of you who are into incense the most sensually pleasurable fragrance I have found is "Indian Rose" which is both exotic and romantic and will remind you of full blown roses in summer. "Indian Rose" is guaranteed to get rid of any un-goddess like smells in your home and is available in most markets and Asian shops.

Smell

9

SMELL & FOOD
& THINGS

"You are what you eat." How many times have we been told that by the experts? It is true, of course and we also *smell* of what we drink and smoke as well as eat: at least our breath, hair and bodies do. Excessive alcohol consumed regularly will be leaked through your pores and you will smell disgusting! Garlic, onions, cabbage and asparagus are some of the more obvious "pongy" foods. Too many vegetables or fruit combined with other foods can lead to flatulence so think carefully about the after effects of everything you eat and drink, especially if you are in a romantic mood.

Smoking is out of the question, of course, and we have already discussed how to get rid of this unhealthy and less than fragrant habit. If you are *still* smoking, I can only say you will have to spend a fortune on breath sprays and perfume to mask the smell. (Unless of course you find a man who smokes, in which case he will not notice your smell as he will have lost his sense of smell to a large extent through smoking and, sadly, so will you if you persist.)

Cooking smells do unfortunately cling so please do not cook in your posh frox and always spray your hair and body with something more appropriate when you remove your apron. You may all want to be domestic goddesses like NIGELLA LAWSON but I am happy to report that The Luscious One is also a truly fragrant woman.

THE CAFÉ DELANCEY described by TIME OUT as *"The Grande Dame of the NW1 eating and drinking scene"* was one of the pioneers of the café/brasserie concept in London. One of my personal favourite restaurants, CAFÉ DELANCEY was as famous for its beautiful and fragrant floral decorations as for its delicious nosh. So I asked

CARLO BERBATOVCI, the CAFÉ's head chef, to prepare a healthy and delicious three course meal which is very fragrant and will *not* make your breath or body stink. CARLO explained that onions do not have any "pongy" effect on your breath or skin once they are cooked until golden and that there is a trick to stopping garlic from smelling too. Read on:

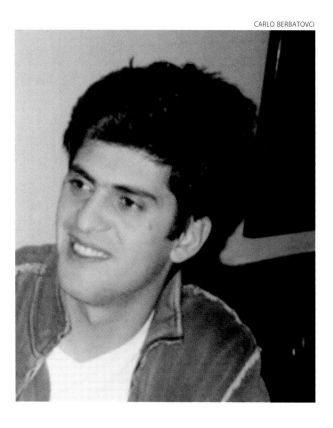

CARLO BERBATOVCI

THREE COURSE FRAGRANT MENU

from Carlo Berbatovci, Café Delancey

Course one: Starter
Green pea soup with mint   *Serves 6*

INGREDIENTS
1 kg peas (frozen or fresh)
500 g potatoes
1 large onion
Fresh mint

METHOD
1 Cover the bottom of the pan with olive oil. Fry chopped onion until golden.
2 Add the peas and potatoes and continue to fry.
3 Add enough water to cover the vegetables, add 2 tbs salt and 1 tbs freshly ground black pepper. Bring to the boil and simmer for one hour.
4 Puree in an electric blender. Fold chopped mint (2 tbs). Check seasoning and serve decorated with a large sprig of mint.

Course two: Main course
Braised lamb shanks   *Serves 6*

INGREDIENTS
6 fresh Welsh lamb shanks
Flour for dredging
Salt and pepper
½ tsp oregano
½ tsp thyme
½ cup olive oil
1 cup each of: chopped onion, chopped carrots, chopped celery
*2 cloves garlic finely chopped *see tip below*
1 cup each of red wine and beef bouillon (gravy)

METHOD
1 In a paper bag, combine flour, salt, pepper, oregano and thyme. Wipe the lamb shanks well, drop one at a time in the paper bag to get them properly coated.
2 Brown them in the oil until golden. Transfer them to an earthenware casserole large enough to take the six side by side.
3 Fry the vegetables for five minutes, add the wine and scrape pan well. Pour the vegetables and wine over the lamb. Add the gravy. Cover and bake for two hours (or until meat is tender) in 350°F.
4 To serve: Stand the lamb shank on the sauce and insert a long stick of dry rosemary inside the hollow bone. Surround with some freshly made mashed potatoes. Decorate with a large sprig of curly fresh parsley.
5 Ignite the rosemary as you bring it to the table. Looks beautiful and the fragrance is superb.

Course three: Dessert
Poached strawberries

A fragrant, delicious sauce to pour over ice cream, sorbet, poached peaches, milk pudding. Keep refrigerated in a jar ready to use

INGREDIENTS
1 kg strawberries (fresh or frozen)
100 g white sugar (less or more according to taste and depending on how sweet the strawberries are)
1 large piece of cinnamon stick
10 cloves

METHOD
1 Cover strawberries with water and bring to the boil.
2 Decrease heat and simmer for five minutes.
3 Remove strawberries.
4 Simmer until water is reduced by a quarter.
5 Pour over strawberries and store or use immediately (cold or hot).

Tips

1 Remove the green shoot inside the clove of garlic by cutting the clove in half – no more complaints about bad breath or indigestion.
2 Fry onions until golden or at least well cooked through
3 Decorate your dishes with raw, clean curly parsley – eat the parsley
4 Chew a coffee bean

Sight

10

BEAUTY
MAKE-UP

"BEAUTY is in the eye of the beholder", so we are told. There is beauty, both inner and outer, in all of us; we just have to find it. Having perfectly symmetrical features is not necessarily it; the much loved PRINCESS DIANA did not have perfect features but she was one of the greatest modern beauties. Do not worry if you are not a naturally blue eyed, rosy cheeked blonde: that can all be fixed with cosmetics and cosmetic aids in today's world. Learn to make the best of yourself, to appreciate your good points and to hide your bad ones. Think yourself beautiful from within and carry yourself like a goddess. Kiss yourself in the mirror every day; nobody else will appreciate you if you do not appreciate yourself.

So how can we make ourselves more kissable, more kiss worthy? Love and success will both give you an inner glow but are sometimes hard to achieve on a permanent basis! But if you eat healthily, exercise, do not smoke and only drink alcohol in moderation you are giving your natural beauty the best possible chance. Your skin, hair and eyes will all shine and you will exude vitality which is highly attractive.

Now we just need to work on the outside. Men do not like us to wear too much make-up but we women know that we look better with at least a lick of paint. The trick is to apply your make-up cunningly so that it looks natural whilst still enhancing your assets. Sadly this takes ages but practice makes perfect. In the evenings and for special occasions we are allowed to go a bit madder with the war paint, the chaps accept it. Anyway we all know that we really apply make-up for each other, not the guys, don't we, ladies?

Face products

Finding the right make-up to suit our individual skins and colouring is seriously confusing with all the products currently available. You only have one face so be careful what you coat it in. If your skin is very sensitive and you are allergic to strong make-up then go for ALMAY or CLINIQUE but all the top cosmetics houses manufacture excellent products which are usually safe for your skin. You cannot go far wrong with CHANEL, DIOR, YSL, LANCÔME, LAUDER, MAC and BOBBI BROWN, all available in the big stores. If you have financial constraints, REVLON, MAX FACTOR and L'ORÉAL are cheaper and are also available in BOOTS, along with all the seriously cheap brands which are useful for experimenting if you are just starting out on the big make-up adventure. Do get your "colours" done at an early stage: for your hair and make-up as well as your wardrobe. COLOUR ME BEAUTIFUL, (66 The Business Centre, 15–17 Ingate Place, London SW8 3NS, phone 020 7627 5211, www.cmb.co.uk) Europe's leading image consultants are simply the best for this vital task. CMB say:

"Whether you are armed with all the latest make-up application techniques or not, the colours of the make-up you wear will either enhance your natural beauty or will…not!

Don't you just get lost when facing a gorgeous looking display of lipsticks? You may even end up buying the latest shade just because it is new. Having bought the most deliciously-packed lipstick, it remains at the bottom of your make-up bag because once you saw yourself wearing it in real day light, it simply didn't do a thing for you.

Lipsticks come in light and dark shades, they come in warm and cool shades, as well as muted and bright colours! What a maze!

Colour consultants are the best to advise what make-up colours are best suited to your natural complexion, eyes and hair combination. To find your nearest Colour Me Beautiful consultant call 020 7627 5211 or visit www.cmb.co.uk. Alternatively, you can find out for yourself which are your best make-up shades in their new book Colour Me Confident *(Hamlyn, February 2006)"*

Colour conscious

Finding the right make-up for you personally requires time and experimentation; that is what testers are for and do not be shy to ask the make-up ladies to help you and even give you a make over when they are not too busy. "No buying without trying" should be your motto when you first start investing in make-up, something which will soon become an ongoing expense, trust me! Each individual's face and skin is different and your skin tone changes as you get older so you will need to change your make-up colours from time to time. However there are some products which every lady needs in her make-up arsenal and the following suit most skin types:

- YSL's "Touche Eclat", currently the best selling make-up product in DEBENHAMS, amongst other shops. This product is great for party girls or for anyone who has ever looked slightly tired (all of us!) There is nothing to touch it for concealing dark rings under the eyes and bringing back the sparkle to a jaded face. In the UK there is just one shade, "Touche Eclat Classic" but overseas you can buy "Touche Eclat 2" for Asian skin and "Touche Eclat 3" for dark skin.
- DIOR's "Diorskin Airflash Mist Make Up which you can spray on and blend in to your skin in ten seconds: a must for the handbag.
- L'ORÉAL's "Cashmere Perfect" liquid powder foundation, the lightest but most covering cheap base I have found or L'ORÉAL's "True Match", a foundation which perfectly adjusts to the colour and texture of your individual skin.
- Any LANCÔME mascara: they are all brilliant but I particularly favour "Hypnose". DIOR's "Diorshow" Backstage Make Up mascara and ESTÉE LAUDER's "Lash XL" are also very good. If you are looking for a cheap alternative, the MAYBELLINE range of mascaras are excellent.
- Recently there was a "mascara revolution" when I.D. BARE ESSENTIALS brought out their amazing "Magic Wand Brushless Mascara". This unusual product allows

you to coat each lash separately for a totally clog free effect and is ideal if you like to use mascara on false lashes (either strip or individual). Phone 0870 850 6655 for stockists.

- MAC's "Powder Blush" is great or, if you prefer a cream, try CLINIQUE's "Cream Blusher".
- MAC'S iridescent powder in "Golden Bronze" for instant sun goddess appeal.
- Any DIOR eye shadow: they are the softest and easiest to apply on the delicate eye area where the skin must *not* be stretched, please, ever! DIOR's "5-Colour Eyeshadow" is a good investment and lasts for ages.
- NOUBA "Rainbow" eye liner (the brightest and most iridescent colours for evening and parties) and NO 17's "Perfect Definition" eye pencil which glides on beautifully, both available from BOOTS.
- REVLON's "Colorstay" lipstick-and-sealer: invest in various colours, this product is quite reasonable and really does have great staying power.

If money is no object go for CHANEL lippies and matching nail polishes: all the colours are jewel bright and goddess like. But you do not have to spend a fortune: The American company, OPI's nail polishes are brilliant and reasonably priced. The OPI lacquers are also much loved by the celeb world including JENNIFER LOPEZ, BRITNEY SPEARS, CHARLIZE THERON, MADONNA, REESE WITHERSPOON, BARBRA STREISAND and literally all the gals with the sexiest talons in the business. You can order the OPI colours from 01923 240 010 or www.lenawhite.co.uk

Over on this side of the pond I recently found a wonderful company called CETUEM whose vitamin E enriched lipsticks and non chipping nail lacquers are excellent and extremely reasonable; available in many stores now and from www.cetuem.com. CETUEM also manufacture the best, lightest and most holding "Finishing Hairspray" (Firm or Natural hold) I have ever come across and that is saying something for a big haired lady such as moi who has tried the lot.

A good collection of brushes for blushing and bronzing and for outlining and blending lips, eyes and brows is also essential. CLINIQUE have a fabulous range which are really soft. But you do not need to buy expensive make-up brushes. TESCO's BARBARA DALY brushes at between £1.00 to £6.00 each are excellent. In fact the whole BARBARA DALY collection at TESCO is superb and the prices are amazing.

We all love a bargain and, apart from TESCO, the cheapest make-up can be found in BOOTS; the BOURJOIS range is particularly good value for youngsters or if you are on a tight budget.

For those of you who like natural products you must try beauty author SIDRA SHAUKAT's "Buff's IncrEdible Edibles" range, especially her divine lip gloss which looks, tastes and smells completely yummy. (Order from: www.sidrashaukat.biz)

Dark skin

If you have dark or black skin you must take care because your skin is more prone to scarring due to its higher pigment. Apply Vitamin E cream or Vitamin E oil locally for scars; these are also excellent for aged and dehydrated skin of any colour and for stretch marks. On the plus side darker skin ages more slowly. The most famous make-up house for black skin is BOBBI BROWN, whose products are all excellent. Celebrated black actress JOAN HOOLEY of *Eastenders*, etc. fame (Anita Arun Representation, phone 020 7379 6840) gave me the benefit of her years of experience trying different make-up and skin care products.

"Black beauty

When I was much younger, and that was a long time ago, finding make-up that suited my dark brown skin was a nightmare. Getting that effortlessly glamorous look that every young woman strives for was extremely elusive.

Black people living in England, until just about ten years ago, struggled to get a natural look as very few of the big names in the world of beauty catered for Caribbean or Afro-Caribbean skins.

In the Television studios, when I was being made up for the very first series I ever worked on, Cool for Cats, *the make-up girls used a greasy pan-stick base, often far too pale for my skin. It clogged the pores. To make matters worse, powders were always too light or too dark and the colour had to be mixed in an attempt to produce a passable result.*

Shades of lipstick were ghastly. My plum red lips didn't appeal. I often created my own colours like a painter with a palette. Things had not improved much in the make-up department when I joined the cast of Emergency Ward 10 in the mid sixties.

However, thankfully those days have long gone. Over the years manufacturers woke up and worked hard to fill the yawning gap in the market place which is now awash with choices for black skins.

At nearly seventy years of age, I can truthfully say that I am now spoilt for choice. Colours in foundations, cleansers, powders, blushers and lipsticks exist in abundance.

It is really not necessary to buy the most expensive product on the market to achieve the best results. What is more

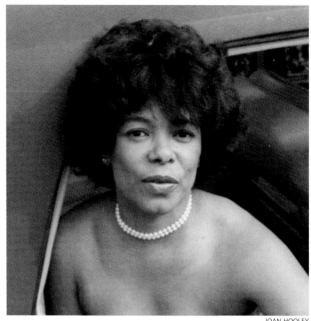
JOAN HOOLEY

important is to develop good habits about caring for your skin. A routine will soon become as automatic as cleaning your teeth or changing your knickers daily!

I am meticulous about cleansing my skin thoroughly at night and use Autopalm Facial Foam Wash or Olay Deep Pore Cleanser, both of which are excellent and affordable. However, I am quite extravagant when it comes to night creams and most of the time splurge on Clarins Raffermissante Nuit which is an extra firming night cream. I have very dry skin and feel that a good night feed makes sense. But I do change my night creams regularly as I am sure that, just as our bodies benefit from change in the foods we eat, so does our skin.

Choosing a foundation is time consuming. I always try several before buying. The texture and consistency is as important as the colour as care has to be taken not to clog the pores with a base that is too heavy. Remember, most ladies apply a foundation in the morning that has to last them throughout the day. Buy the best quality that you can afford. The same goes for the power you use.

Take time and effort to apply both carefully. Always apply make-up in a good light as streaks, specially on a dark sin, are most unattractive. Apply your powder quite generously. I use Clinique 06 Glow. Pat gently onto the face, and use a good quality brush to remove excess: Try MAC Tapered Blending Brush 222 or Clinique Powder Brush, a sleek handmade brush which has a unique, anti-microbial technology to prevent it from growing mould, fungus and bacteria – which can happen particularly if you store your brushes in the bathroom as I do. A good brush helps you to achieve a flawless finish.

Allow ample time for make-up! Whatever your age, time spent on your make-up reflects the care you have taken to make yourself look great at the start of the day. Surely that's what every woman wants. I certainly do.

Shu Uemura Blending Brush 20BL is great for applying well-defined shadows or creating killer cheekbones. Never apply too much blusher to the cheeks. They should look subtly sun-kissed and not as if you are on your way to an Indian war paint party!

Don't forget your lips. Smear on the Vaseline whenever they feel slightly rough or chapped. Believe me it works, leaving you with soft kissable lips. I have never found anything better and so cheap.

Start caring for your skin at an early age. Although most black people have been blessed with great skin, don't neglect it. You will certainly reap the benefits as you grow older and you will be glad you followed the advice of an OAP who looks great for her age.

And for heaven's sake, don't linger in the sun too long. Many people are of the opinion that black people never get sunburnt. This is not true. I was badly sunburnt as a teenager. A painful experience."

ASIAN SKIN

If you are Asian, you are lucky; you probably have beautiful skin! Here Indian TV star RANI SINGH talks us through make-up and hair for (South) Asian ladies.

Make-up and hair

(South) Asians love spending money on make-up and more and more manufacturers have woken up to the power of the brown pound. In theory, we are fortunate in that our skin tones can easily take bright lipstick colours like fuchsia, pink or red – we can also enjoy wearing shades of gold on the eyes, lips and cheeks. However there are some points to bear in mind.

However much water I drink and however much oxygen I breathe, there is nothing like a facial to deep cleanse the skin occasionally.

For **foundation**, remember to try it out on the jaw line not the back of the hand; as liquid can oxidise do wait a bit before making a purchase.

For the fairest of our skin types I would recommend La Prairie, Almay and Shiseido, moving to Bobbi Brown, Mac, Prescriptives, Clinique and Lancôme for darker tones.

(South) Asian skin has a tendency to look sallow in winter so to counteract this, blend **bronzers** with **blushers** under the cheekbones. Good blushers to use are Pin Ya Cheeks Cheek Stain, Clinique's cream blusher; Dior is great too.

For Bronzers, try Clarins, Guerlain, Marks and Spencer and Origins' Picture Cheeks.

While my make-up artists tell me that golds tend to suit me best, more experimental colours for brown eyes are yellow, green, lilac and blue. Try pink if you have green eyes.

Kohl was invented by and for us in the first instance, and I wear it inside my lower lids (try green or blue kohl with brown eyes too). I use liquid black eyeliner on my upper lid, but it's hard to find eyeliners which stay smooth and which don't sting if they run into the eyes. Mac is good for eyeliner and mascara.

(South) Asian eyes can be prone to dark circles so remedy this with either the Mac or the Kanebo eye circle concealer. Cobalt blue, grey and mulberry-toned mascara can draw attention away from dark circles too.

With bright eye make-up, keep the **lips** sheer and glossy. Max Factor's Lipfinity is great for nude lips. A tip for those with thin lips; dark colours make them look thicker. I hate going without lipstick and glossies are my favourite. Yves Saint Laurent, Shiseido, Nars and Shu Uemura have some lovely vibrant lip colours. Guerlain's lip lift, put on first underneath the colours helps staying power and avoids bleeding.

(South) Asian beauticians advise us to bleach, wax or electrolyse any facial hair, as ours tends to be dark and they like us to have a smooth-looking face before applying make-up. Threading, where cotton thread is weaved between the beautician's fingers and used to remove the hair quickly, is the cheapest method of dealing with the problem, and is now quite common in UK salons.

While (South) Asian make-up has to be specific to our needs, no discussion of make-up can be complete without talking about **hair** as the two need to complement each other.

Our hair is quite different to European hair as it is mostly darker, thicker and more porous. Generally speaking, our hair can tolerate more chemicals as well, though if the scalp is sensitive, then chemical-free and ammonia-free options are always available. Hair conditioning treatments like warm oil are very useful.

I need versatile styles which are easy to manage so senior stylist and London College of Fashion graduate Nahren Yalda keeps changing my hair colour and style according to work demands; presenting serious current affairs documentaries requires a different style to children's television!

Nahren's clients are European, Mediterranean, Middle Eastern and South Asian. So she is well versed in our needs. She advises that, because our skin tones tend to be darker, one-colour hair should be avoided. Warm hair colours, lowlights and highlights can lift skin tones and bring out the colours of the eyes.

It is important to change the hairstyle to find a version which keeps us looking contemporary while finding something which suits our faces. In my case, short hair works best. For South Asians, wild, crazy colours don't really suit us.

We have a gorgeous cultural legacy of ornaments apart from earrings and necklaces to wear around the face and in the hair to complement our make-up. We have our nose jewels (stick-on ones go nicely at the side of the nose for a pain-free temporary fashion accessory) as well as beautiful bejewelled clips to wear at the side of the hair or down a centre parting. Wearing these makes me feel very regal and special.

I include "bindis"* in make-up and have lots on my dressing table. They are now so popular that few self-respecting international female pop stars appear in their music videos without one decorating their foreheads. I always put on a bindi if I'm going to a party and "Jazzy Bindi" do some fantastic and unique designs. Their latest ones are pure silver, hand crafted and plated in rodium, 22 or 18 carat gold! Such a special item placed on the forehead for a few hours can really make you feel like a million dollars and is the perfect finale to any make-up session!

*"Bindis" are the decorative symbol placed in the middle of a married lady's forehead; its tradition and history is religious but now it is a must-have fashion item, and teenagers and women all over the world have them. Singles like me love them to bits as we can get any shade or design to match our outfits and mood. We stick them on with special glue and "Jazzy Bindi" sell exclusive designer ones. By tradition it was a red little circle but now we can have them any colour or colours, sometimes several bindis can be worn at once to make up a little pattern.

Contacts: Nahren Yalda (mobile 07958 355 531), Top salon director at **Peach on the Hill**, 140 Campden Hill Road, Kensington, London W8 7AS..

Jazzy Bindi, phone 020 8471 7457.

Make-up tips

If you have never worn make-up before, either because you are very young or because make-up is just not your thing but suddenly you are expected to wear some for a big occasion, do not panic. You can always have a session or two with a professional make-up artiste who will advise you on colours and types of make-up for your particular face and skin.

Certainly it is advisable to book a make-up artiste for a really special occasion, such as your wedding day, to bring out the true goddess in you. For a start it is much more relaxing to be made up by somebody else and you will feel totally pampered and gorgeous. Here top make-up artiste DANIELLE RENSHAW (07855 958 682, www.ivoventuri.com) who works regularly with the excellent RMK COSMETICS, gives you a few pointers.

MAKE-UP TIPS
from Danielle Renshaw

1 Prepare skin. **Exfoliate and moisture** masque once a week while cleansing, toning and moisturising AM and PM and don't forget the eye cream! Good make-up starts with good skin!

2 For a healthy summer glow use **self tan**. Sun products are amazing!

3 Apply a **make-up base**, which will make the foundation last all day, look even on the skin, and balance oiliness of skin throughout the day!

4 Use a light **concealer** if necessary, around the eyes (lids as well as under), as well as on any spots! *Tip*: nostrils tend to redden so add a little around them.

5 Choose a light, dewy finish **foundation**. Check in daylight for best results to determine the colour and apply with wet sponge, foundation brush or fingers! I love RMK's liquid foundation, it's water-resistant and contains SPF 15, and with a fresh, dewy finish it's fab for summer!

6 **Powder** if you tend to be more on the oily T zone side or if you feel the foundation is a little sticky, use a powder that will give you a bit of a luminous glow like YSL's Poudre Sur Mesure or RMK's PO2 Powder brush on.

7 **Eyes** these days are very easy; you can even apply with your fingers! Creamy shades of emerald greens, metallic golds and turquoise blues are applied effortlessly by pressing the pigment onto lid all over eye. Try YSLs' Fard Eclat liquid waterproof shadow, to die for! Girls with blue and green eyes try greens and blues as they will bring out your natural colour. In corner of eye (the crease) add a darker colour (greys, chocolate browns), and blend with finger or a blending brush inwards to the centre of the eye. This will add some depth to the colour used all over, great for nights out! You can if you want to achieve the "smoky eye" apply a black or charcoal powder as close as you can along the lash line with a liner brush. The powder will stick to the cream and look not as harsh as if you were to use a pencil. Looking good!
Brown-eyed girls have it easy; they can just about get away with every colour, so experiment with it! Metallic colours look and feel amazing to use or try to add some pink with grey, very effective!

8 Curl **eyelashes** and apply mascara, one application looks natural; two, with another curl, really opens the eye area!

9 Brush **brows** with brow comb or even a toothbrush and apply brow gel or a little Vaseline to make them stay in place.

10 **Bronzer** is a nice touch if you don't like using self-tan. It will accentuate the sun kissed parts of the face, use with a powder brush on cheekbones, sides of forehead, temples, bridge of nose, chin and décolleté.

11 Creamy **cheek** colours are a very natural way to give colour to the cheeks. Apply with fingers on the apple of the cheek and blend with fingers or sponge. Start with minimal and add to it if needed.

12 Last but not least, **lips**! Juicy non-sticky glosses are available and also sheer moisture sticks are in for the season; try to match the same hues with the blush. Corals look great on a tanned skin and pinks look nice on a bronzed skin. Spritz skin to set the make-up with one of RMK's herb mists and you're ready to go! Tip; brush lips day and night with toothbrush for exfoliated, soft bee stung lips!

Danielle Renshaw has been making up faces for twelve years. Originally from Vancouver, BC, she worked in fashion, film and television, which gained her a vast creative knowledge of colour and technique. Arriving in London three years ago, Danielle uses her skills and creative flair, freelancing and working with RMK cosmetics. To book in with Danielle for a consultation please ring 07855 958 682 or website ivoventuri.com. Hope to meet you soon!

Hair products

Getting back to special occasions, it goes without saying that you should have your hair done professionally as well as your make-up. Celebrity make-up and hair artiste and stylist to the stars SHARON BLACK (07767 296690) who has made me up for various TV and newspaper shoots advises "always leave enough time to achieve the total look: hair, make-up, clothes, accessories".

We all have to learn to look after our hair ourselves and there is a plethora of wonderful products out there in all the pharmacies. However if we are talking hair health it is probably safest to buy professional hair products from hair salons; for instance you cannot go wrong with the wonderful NICKY CLARKE range. NICKY CLARKE has salons in Birmingham and Manchester but his flagship salon is at 130 Mount Street, W1K 3NY, phone 020 7491 4700 where you can buy his products in person or order over the phone. NICKY's "Blonde Goddess Colour Therapy" range will definitely make your tresses feel goddess like, especially the "See Me/Colour and Shine" shampoo. The charming NICKY, who is himself an excellent advert for his products and services, says his personal favourites are:

- ❧ "60 Second Secret" conditioner, his biggest selling conditioner and most successful hair care product,
- ❧ "Creme de Luxe", the finishing product which he uses on 90% of his clients and says is great for the majority of styles including straight, curly and choppy and
- ❧ "Hair Raising", his favourite body building product (which reminds me of the famous quote about blonde goddess FARRAH FAWCETT MAJORS, "her hair has more body than her body": no doubt your hair will too after using "Hair Raising").

The GOLDWELL range is also superb and is available at loads of hair salons (or "hair saloons" as the legendary *How to Marry A Millionaire* director, BILLY CARTER likes to call them!) GOLDWELL TRENDLINE manufacture fab mousses, waxes and sprays including their "Extreme Shine/Shine Spray" which is great for enlivening dull hair. Their CARE range includes some terrific shampoos and conditioners and, if you are brave enough to colour your own hair, try their "Colour Glow" range. My personal GOLDWELL favourite is their "Golden Spray" hairspray which does the business on big hair every time.

REDKEN is another excellent range for all sorts of hair products which can be purchased at most salons. Their "Airtight Lock-Out Finishing Spray" was one of my "Products of the Month" at HOT GOSSIP recently. It is a hair spray which actually protects your hair against rain and damp and humid conditions, an absolute must for many European climates, not to mention Florida.

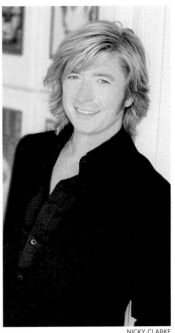

NICKY CLARKE

Sight

II

BEAUTY
SKIN CARE

Skin care is a very important consideration. It is never too early to start nourishing your skin and protecting it from the elements. If you are very young with perfect skin you can get away with using just a moisturiser: NIVEA is great for young skins. As you get older, however, you will need to use nourishing cream at night and bring out the big guns to prevent and get rid of wrinkles. If your skin is dry I suggest you start your nourishing regime from an earlier age than your oily skinned sisters: probably in your twenties or as soon as you spot the first tell-tale signs of ageing.

Skin care products
Your cleansing and toning routine is also of paramount importance, especially after wearing make-up and if you live in a big dirty city like London. If you have acne or spots of any kind it is even more important to keep the skin clean and fresh to avoid the spread of the dreaded zits! A good product for young skin is ST IVES' "Apricot Scrub" cleanser, available at BOOTS, which comes in various formats for different skin types including "blemish control".

CLINIQUE's product range is all clinically formulated, allergy tested and 100% fragrance free so is ideal for young and/or troubled skins. Their "Anti-blemish Solutions" Cleansing Foam and Concealing Stick are particularly effective. CLINIQUE's "Super Defense" range is also excellent for all ages. For more mature skin try their "Dramatically Different Moisturising Lotion" which has a handy pump dispenser and "Advanced Stop Signs Eye" eye cream.

All the top cosmetics houses manufacture amazing cleansing, toning and nourishing products, as well as creams and serums to prevent and get rid of wrinkles. My personal favourites (for my middle-aged skin) among the big houses are LANCÔME and ESTÉE LAUDER, all of whose products are superb. I also use CLARINS' famous "Beauty Flash Balm" from time to time to brighten and tighten my skin when it looks dull. New skin care companies and products are being launched all the time; it is a good idea to try everything until you find out what suits you best. Your skin also gets used to certain products after a while and they may become less effective, in which case you will need to rotate your different favourites.

Cosmetic doctor DR PATRICK BOWLER has recently brought out a new range of anti-ageing products, exclusive to him, called "Vitage". The range includes "Smooth Lines" which is self-explanatory and "Even Tones" which combats uneven pigmentation, age spots and so on without causing undue skin irritation. You can order these products from 0870 850 6655.

SKIN DOCTORS is a British company who are best known for manufacturing PERFECT POUT, a lip plumping product which really works. I particularly favour their RELAXADERM or "Botox in a jar" which prevents facial expressions from forming wrinkles and ANTARCTILYNE, a rich "plumping up" cream with a secret ingredient from the Antarctic Ocean which you apply after the RELAXADERM to achieve smooth, youthful looking skin.

SKIN DOCTORS also produce excellent acne and spot treating products, including their BLEMISHFREE pack of medicated cleanser, toner, pore reduction cream and ZIT ZAPPER, a self explanatory wand product which is a must for getting rid of the odd pimple within hours: "don't leave home without it"! SKIN DOCTORS' products are available from BOOTS and major department stores nationwide or ring 0800 298 9600 for your nearest stockist.

DR DENESE is another excellent (American) skin care company recently launched on these shores. The eponymous DR D is a truly stunning lady in her fifties who looks twenty years younger: talk about setting a good example! The DR DENESE range of products (01295 72 45 83, www.drdenese.co.uk) is superb and reasonably priced and includes a "Home Microdermabrasion Kit" which is a truly brilliant idea that I use myself. Other good investments from this range are their "Hydroseal Hand and Décolleté Serum", "Line-Erase" and "Retinol Max Capsules". Their "Vitamin C Radiance Cream" which is chock full of nourishing vitamins and ceramides is a marvellous invention which literally fills in fine lines and wrinkles, especially around the mouth and eyes. You apply it underneath your foundation and it gives you an instant flawless finish which feels really silky to the touch. I love it myself and really miss its effect if I forget to put it on by mistake!

According to DR DENESE, celebrity fans of the range include SADIE FROST, LISA SNOWDEN, MARIELLA FROSTRUP and JODIE KIDD.

For those of you who have problems with redness, general discoloration and flakiness try ESTÉE LAUDER's "Idealist Skin Refinisher" which improves the colour, tone and texture of your skin within weeks.

If you like to take your anti-ageing products orally or to give your nourishing regime an extra boost, you must try PURELOGICOL's "Age-defying Body Supplement" capsules made from pure collagen; remember "beauty comes from within". In fact the PURELOGICOL range is excellent for anti-ageing. They manufacture a superb "Age Defying Face Mask" with pure collagen which should be used once a week ideally and the PURELOGICOL "Age Defying Velvet Face Serum" with pure collagen is absolute magic for mature skin.

Do not leave your mouth out of your moisturising and nourishing regime. The delicate skin of the mouth is fragile and lips are the first area to dry out when the elements are rough. Carry a lip care stick with you at all times, especially if you use drying "stay fast" lipsticks: all the BOOTS lipsalves are fine but the richest is definitely CROOK's "E45" lipsalve. One of the best and cheapest of these products is TESCO's "Lip Smoother" which is also a convenient stick product. (TESCO's "Make-up Eye-lift" is another little gem from this range which you can dab on at any time when you are not wearing make-up.)

For those of you who like to buy products for all the family ORANGEBURST's new "Skinfood" range of cleansers, moisturisers, masques and scrubs is suitable for ladies, gents and kids. The products are based on natural ingredients such as Manuka honey, coconut palm, aloe vera, avocado oil, lavender oil and essential orange and contain no artificial colourings or fragrance. They are all very reasonably priced and are available from leading health food stores or from 01273 558 112, www.lemonburst.net

If you want to go the all-natural route there is a new Aloe Vera range called FOREVER LIVING PRODUCTS whose moisturisers, sunscreens, shampoos, soap etc. are really pure and wholesome and which feel great on the skin. The extensive range includes make-up and health drinks and supplements as well as skin care. I particularly like the FOREVER deodorant stick which "contains no aluminium salts": spraying or rubbing aluminium into your armpits with other products is certainly not a healthy option. If only we knew precisely what was in all the products we plaster on ourselves every day and if only we had time in our busy lives to read the fine print on the labels! It is certainly a good idea to use natural products if you can find them. The FOREVER range is sold through distributors and can be mail ordered; my lady who is extremely friendly and helpful is PAM TAYLOR (07985 432236).

Dermatologists

If you have serious skin problems of any kind you may need to see a dermatologist. DR PENELOPE TYMPANIDIS is a Consultant Dermatologist who heads up the RENASCENCE "Facial Aesthetics" clinic (19 Wimpole Street, London, W1G 8GE, phone 020 7462 0030, www.renascence.co.uk). DR TYMPANIDIS is best known on TV ("EXTREME MAKE OVERS", etc.) and in the media for her anti-ageing treatments but she knows everything there is to know about skin in general. Here is her report:

SKIN CONDITIONS

from Dr Penelope Tympanidis

Acne

Patients suffering from acne need to undergo a proper dermatological assessment by a consultant dermatologist.

Apart from teenage acne there is increasing incidence of late onset acne, which may occur in the twenties or even thirties. Polycystic ovaries and/or other hormonal depending conditions might trigger acne.

Treatment will include chemical peeling, and topical preparations application to start with. With these, not only do I aim to treat acne *per se*, but I also try to treat or minimise the post acne scarring.

Acne of mild degree may respond to topical treatment only.

For acne of moderate to severe degree, I consider systemic treatment alongside peeling and topical preparations.

The first line systemic treatment comprises antibiotics, most of the time tetracycline. In cases of stubborn "hormone" depended acne some physicians may combine oral contraceptives combined with antibiotics.

I am not in favour of this approach and prefer to prescribe an all natural remedy, comprising hormones coming from the plants, so called phyto-oestrogens. These do not have the side effects of the oral contraceptive pill but may be as beneficial.

Should this prove to be ineffective, I consider, based on the clinical severity and extent of acne, treatment with Roaccutane.

Roaccutane is retinoic acid (pro-vitamin A) in the form of tablets, and the course lasts 4–6 months. It is a prescription-only tablet suitable for severe acne vulgaris. Patients on Roaccutane should be closely followed up by the dermatologist, and undergo blood tests before, during and after the course of treatment as it may affect their liver function. Women of child-bearing age should not get pregnant during the treatment with Roaccutane.

However Roaccutane in most cases has been proven to be a "miracle" drug for severe stubborn acne.

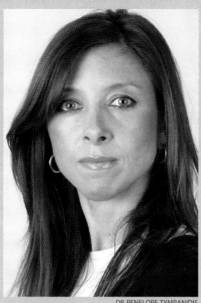

DR PENELOPE TYMPANIDIS

In my practice I also deal a lot with post acne scarring.

This may be a long laborious process comprising chemical peeling of various strengths and types, scar remodelling and undermining as well as topical preparations application.

Warts

Warts and veruccas are a very common viral skin condition. The wart virus is ubiquitous, therefore anybody may get them.

Genital warts are sexually transmitted. If a woman gets genital warts she should immediately see a dermatologist for treatment.

This is because if genital warts spread trough the vagina, they may affect the cervix. If the cervix is affected by genital warts, this is considered a pre-cancerous condition, which might develop into cervical cancer. This is why, in the event of genital warts on a female patient, immediate treatment by a dermatologist and a smear test by a gynaecologist is mandatory.

I usually treat warts and veruccas with cryotherapy (freezing with liquid nitrogen treatment) and/or topical preparations such as salicylic acid.

There is a novel compound Imiquimod, which is proven to be effective on warts in the form of cream. The old fashioned topical treatment with Formaldehyde is often effective but patients have to be cautious, as Formaldehyde can be noxious for the skin.

Actinic ageing/skin cancer

Many patients visit me for their sun-damaged skin. Due to the ozone hole, the sun has become extremely aggressive and there is no doubt that extensive sun exposure will cause premature ageing of the skin, and increase the incidence of skin cancer. Cases of melanoma have multiplied greatly in the last few years. Therefore application of sun block when exposed to the sun is mandatory.

People with fair skin are more prone to actinic damage and are those who more often present, already in their fifties, small rodent ulcers, which is a type of benign skin cancer.

The brown spots of the sun-exposed areas (face, back of hands, cleavage), which appear on the skin of individuals who have had extensive sun exposure throughout their lifetime, are due to the cumulative effects of the sun. These brown lesions may be treated with peels, and lasers. With both these forms of treatment the treated areas soon blend in with the rest of the skin.

Although the sun is good for our Vitamin D levels, and good mood, its ultra violet rays are dangerous; you should always moderate your exposure to the sun and wear a sunscreen with a high SPF or a complete sun block.

Some ladies like to have skin tags and moles removed. Skin tags can easily be snipped off then cauterised but moles need to be properly assessed and histologically labelled following excision for reasons of safety.

Vitiligo

Vitiligo is a relatively common autoimmune condition, which may be triggered by stress. Often there is another autoimmune process in the background (i.e. thyroiditis). It is a self-limiting condition therefore may resolve spontaneously. However its course cannot be predicted. It may respond to treatment with topical steroids in the form of cream, steroid injections or even tablets. The latest topical ointment, which has proved successful for mild cases of Vitiligo, is Tacrolimus.

Some cases respond to ultraviolet light therapy in conjunction with application of photosensitive preparations. However this may only take place in specialised centres under close supervision of the dermatologist.

Anti-ageing/Rejuvenation

I have a special interest in anti-ageing and rejuvenation. As a dermatologist in charge at RENASCENCE I offer the cutting edge of all the minimally invasive rejuvenating treatments. I usually assess my patients carefully and personalise their individual skin rejuvenation treatment by "picking and mixing" various techniques and treatments.

The result is a healthier better-looking skin. The aim is to make my patients look their best for their age, without altering their facial features, but restoring their skin condition, facial and body contours.

Chemical peeling is the front line of skincare. There is a huge range of peeling agents and a large range of different strengths of those. Therefore there is the right cocktail of peeling agents for every type of skin: young skin prone to acne spots, sensitive skin, aged or sun damaged skin, etc.

Who Is a candidate?

If you have:
- Superficial wrinkles of the face, neck, upper chest, arms, etc.
- Deep facial wrinkling.
- Uneven pigmentation problems caused by sun exposure, prescription drugs or disease.
- Enlarged facial pores.
- Superficial acne scars of the face.
- "Age spots."

Intended result

Smoother, youthful appearing skin of more uniform colour.

Procedure description

These procedures are done on an outpatient basis. Light peels may be done without any anaesthesia. Light and medium depth peels do not require any anaesthesia.
- After preparing the skin, a series of solutions may be applied.
- Light, moderate or deep peels are available. A consultation is required to determine which type of peel (if any) will be most suitable for you.
- Mesotherapy on the face in the form of microinjections of hyaluronic acid,
- Vitamins and antioxidants may give a healthy glow to the skin and are a very popular anti-ageing treatment.
- Mesotherapy applied on the body is an excellent way of treating cellulite and improving body contours.

In Renascence I have pioneered by introducing SubQ, a novel type of Hyaluronic acid applied as a subcutaneous implant (under the skin close to the bony structures and not into the skin). This is applied for facial sculpturing, for enhancing the chin, the facial contours and cheekbones. With this method I place the filler under the skin close to the bony structures (and not into the skin like most fillers) to give a very subtle and natural look to the cheekbones, hence giving a discreet "lift" to the face.

SubQ is a form of hyaluronic acid which is an extremely safe compound included in the fillers I apply for lip sculpturing and wrinkle remodelling.

I also offer Isolagen live cells rejuvenation therapy. In brief, with this very sophisticated method, I harvest your own fibroblasts (your skin repair cells) expand them and re-inject them into your skin where it needs to be repaired most.

Botox is another popular rejuvenation technique. Despite a lot of misleading press on this, Botox remains one of the safest and most popular procedures. I advise you to be properly informed by a physician before you undergo this. You should also accept treatment by a medical specialist only and not by a non-medical person.

Fillers may improve your looks greatly.

Again seek treatment by a physician with a lot of experience.

Non-permanent non-animal fillers are the safest ones. This is because our skin is a very dynamic organ; it changes all the time and implanting something permanent in it might have a long-term negative outcome.

The most effective and safe fillers are poly-lactic acid, so-called sculptra (excellent for deep lines) and Hyaluronic acid (best for lips and fine lines).

As I said before, "prevention is better than cure" where your skin is concerned. My advice to patients is to go outdoors sensibly, not in the midday sun, seek the shade and always wear a high SPF or sun block in the sun. The core of skin care is not cleansing, toning and nourishing but exfoliation and sun block. I favour chemical peels and can assure you that there is a suitable type of peel for everybody.

Smoking is the worst thing you can do to your skin as it damages the Fibroblasts, which replace the natural collagen and hyaluronic acid of your skin.

Do try to drink alcohol as little as possible or not at all.

Drink lots of water and freshly squeezed juices and eat well. The simple Mediterranean diet is best: grilled meat or fish with loads of fresh vegetables and fruit and olive oil for cooking. Avoid fried foods, over complicated recipes and complex carbohydrates. Then your skin will be as good as it can be.

Skin care

Now let's hear from dewy skinned Indian TV star RANI SINGH as she lets us in to a few of her skin care secrets:

"Our skins are like a shop window for what is inside us; if we are full of tension, chemicals, toxins and the wrong types of food and drink, the skin is where it all shows up.

We can learn a lot from ancient Indian techniques which were laid down in texts 5,000 years ago and many of which are practised round the world today. There are many olden references to Ayurveda, a holistic approach to skincare, diet and the body which encompasses the spiritual as well as the physical. In South Asian culture, it is the whole person who is being treated, so our health and skincare professionals make individual 'prescription treatments' combining physical therapies to soothe and relax muscles, and more esoteric therapies to balance the spirit and mind.

Our ancient texts describe oil massages for the hair and the body and the importance of taking time to deal with the stress of life by relaxation. In India, massage is endemic so it's routine to get someone to come over to your house and very easy to find beauty salons offering this treatment. While working 24/7 in studios in London (for example spending three years on EastEnders) stress can accumulate in the shoulders and neck and this can be detrimental to the skin, as blood circulation is affected and toxins accumulate. So I look to my own cultural history to prevent any skincare problems later on.

The best practitioner I have found to work with me is London-based Brenda Elvin, who treats me (and members of my family) on a regular basis. Massage is necessary when coping with a

RANI SINGH

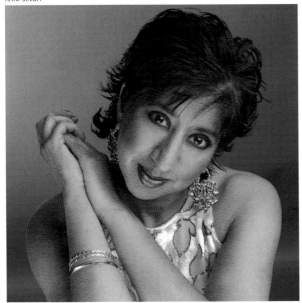

©JOHN DAWSON

schedule where I can be working very intensively, pumping lots of adrenalin round my body preparing to compete at screen tests and performing on camera. I take an Indian head massage from Brenda which stimulates the circulation to scalp and to hair, helps to maintain what people describe as 'a healthy glow', and eases tight neck muscles or an aching head. She uses mixes of oils, and likes me to put Almond oil and also Rosemary oil on my scalp to condition it, just like my ancestors did centuries ago! Indian Head Massage also incorporates acupressure points on the face to help tighten skin and ease tension around the eyes and jaw.

Brenda uses the more 'western' therapy of Swedish and sports massage too, practising deep muscle release techniques which help to keep muscle tissue healthy.

(Interestingly, at the studios of many long running drama series nowadays, there are masseurs who regularly visit, treating actors and other staff.)

Ancient Indians talk about the 'Chakra' system or energy centres around the body and Brenda combines Chakra work with the Japanese Reiki technique which uses hand positions held just above the body to channel energy, to calm and to heal. If my stomach gets tight with anxiety, Brenda works on the Sacral Chakra just above my naval to calm me. It helps to normalise breathing and having the right amount of oxygen going round my body ultimately makes my skin look better.

Ayurveda advocates the use of natural ingredients and methods, and much of South Asian skincare still relies on the technique.

My mother Parsan was a beauty queen in London but she made sure that while I was growing up in the city I kept my skincare quite natural and avoided make-up and chemicals for as long as I could.

For a thorough body scrub she would make a mix of yellow gram flour, oil and turmeric.

A face mask was made up of yoghurt, oats and honey.

And when I started working in film she taught me to always take off my make-up at night, to cleanse and to moisturise.

I also like to drink water and tend to avoid smoky environments if I can although on a film set there are always smokers – often they are other actors!

Brenda Elvin's contact details: 020 8575 8839 and brendaelvin@tiscali.co.uk".

Another lady who knows a thing or two about beauty and advocates the totally natural approach (shock horror!) is mature beauty LYDIA M. SILVESTRY (www.lydiasilvestry.com). A renowned journalist and fashion designer, best known for her patented creation the INFINITE DRESS – a dress that can be changed into over 100 different styles – and author of *My Beauty Secrets*, LYDIA advises:

NATURAL CARE
from Lydia Silvestry

Would you like a lively body and radiant skin? Do you desire a healthy, youthful life? They are yours if you want them. All you need is the knowledge, awareness, and desire. With information from books such as this one you can gain the first two. Combine those with desire, which you must supply yourself, and you shall get there!

Quite regularly I am asked: "How do you keep looking so young?" I have two sons, both approaching their 40s. On countless occasions people, upon seeing me with one or both of my sons, assumed that I was a sister. (Sometimes they later confess they thought I was a younger sister.) When told I am the mother, their first reaction is usually a laugh with an incredulous comment such as "sure!" or "right!" At those moments it then it took a bit of convincing before they accepted that we were not joking, but in fact telling the truth.

Herein I am pleased to share with you a few of my health and beauty secrets. One of the keys to my beauty secrets is replacement: the replacement of chemicals and toxins lurking in your environment that accelerate your ageing with natural ingredients that promote and prolong good living. While it is not possible to completely eliminate all harsh ageing ingredients from your environment, there IS much you can do to limit or diminish their effect on your health and beauty. Through simple replacement you can take important steps toward achieving youthful looks, exuberance and a long exciting life.

My greatest wish is that these simple secrets will inspire you to develop physical, mental and spiritual knowledge and awareness, and that you will convert that knowledge and awareness into a great level of beauty and health that awaits you.

Enjoy a beautiful life!

Secrets for Youthful Hair
Point 1: Your Natural Hair Colour is Beautiful; Hair Dyes Have Harsh Chemicals

Do you colour your hair? If you do then you know that your hair may look good for a few days, but soon thereafter the natural hair will grow out again. Meanwhile, your body is battling against foreign substances that penetrate your scalp. The chemicals in the colouring find their way into your bloodstream, taxing your immune system, causing you to tire more quickly.

Are you still colouring your hair? If so, I ask you to stop at once! Be proud of your true hair colour. Be true to yourself and the world. Let your natural hair colour be a shining example of the real you. Your health and your spirit will show you their appreciations.

Point 2: Use the Earth's Natural Shampoo Rather Than Artificial Chemicals
Great varieties of shampoos come in assorted fragrances from assorted chemical ingredients. Shampoo, unfortunately, is the end product of a process that is anything but natural. While perhaps it is not as powerfully toxic as hair dye, nonetheless, it has many chemical ingredients that are not healthy.

What natural product can you use as substitute for shampoo? Borax. Borax is a natural product packaged in a box "straight" from the earth with no chemical processing or additives. In an empty glass jar or other clean container, pour about one inch of 100% Borax powder, then fill the jar with water. Shake it to dissolve the Borax as much as possible. Now use this liquid mixture to wash your hair. Be aware that it will not form a lather (you get used to this quickly). However, it does leave your scalp and hair clean.

Also use it on your body as a substitute for chemically-laden soap.

Other Hair Points for Your Knowledge and Awareness
- Natural Hair Sprays – lemon juice; castor oil with essential oil
- Natural Hair Glows – olive oil; sesame oil; coconut oil; jojoba oil.
- Natural Hair Conditioners – sesame oil; olive oil; avocado
- Natural Hair Rinse – vinegar; lemon juice; chamomile tea

Secrets for Youthful Skin
Dry skin is the condition about which I hear most women complain. A healthy radiant face is a beautiful face. You can have a radiant face once you diminish and limit the chemicals that lurk in your environment.

For a radiant, healthy face, clean your face with olive oil. If you are still using cosmetics, extra light olive oil is a great make-up remover, mascara remover, and eye shadow remover that your skin will appreciate. For a nice bouquet, add a few drops of aromatherapy to olive oil: lavender, lemon, jasmine, citrus, Ylang Ylang or whatever your favourite may be.

Use olive oil to bathe as well. You will not smell like salad dressing, trust me! Just add the same essential oil described above that you enjoy and you will soon see the results of such regular showers: a glowing skin and lots of fun!

Olive oil is without a doubt one of the most beneficial ingredients that keeps my skin glowing.

Carefully Selected Clothing: Dress for Beautiful Health
About Fabrics
Clothing attire made from man-made fabrics affects your body. It emits a continuous shock to the nerve endings that cover your skin. The electrical charge is subtle but measurable. This affects your youthfulness and beauty, not to mention your nervous system.

You should wear only attire that is conducive to good health and beauty: clothing that is made with natural fibres: 100% cotton, linen, silk, wool, alpaca, cashmere, rayon.

Just as important as the material comprising your clothing is how you wash your clothes. It doesn't help to have 100% natural fabric and then wash it with harmful chemical detergents that stick to the fabric. As a natural laundry detergent use Borax, baking soda, or a combination of the two in small amounts as they are very powerful.

Rinsing: use one cup of vinegar when there are large amounts of stain or mould on the fabric, or for a smooth finish.

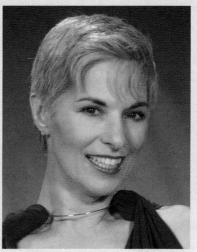

LYDIA SILVESTRY

Secrets to a Healthy Mind

While you will certainly enhance your beauty and health through the techniques described above, for maximum benefit you should simultaneously develop yourself from the inside. Daily meditation is excellent for health-enhancing peace of mind. Through meditation I receive the answers to all my questions. At times the responses are startling, even shocking. However, through the years I have learned to accept the messages as real miracles. To this I attribute the clarity and power of my beauty secrets. When you come down to it, it is simply listening to God.

Sight

12

BEAUTY TREATMENTS

FACE, HAIR & BODY

I F you have the time and the money you should spoil yourself with regular beauty treatments by salon professionals. Facials, massages, hair dos, etc. will all perk you up and bring out the goddess in you. Regular facials and massages will ensure that your skin is in tip top condition all over and of course you must have your hair cut, coloured and conditioned professionally every few weeks even if you can do it yourself brilliantly. For me beauty treatments are absolute bliss and even better stress busters than retail therapy!

What is available

The right age to start having beauty treatments is when you personally are ready. If you are a teenager with bad skin it is a good idea to have regular facials at a good salon. One therapist I have found who is particularly caring and looks at treating the skin in a totally holistic way is CARINA COEN. Irish born CARINA has three MERCARINA clinics but her private clinic (Mercarina Private Clinic, 56 Seymour Street, London, W1, phone 020 7724 0514, www.mercarina.com) is the best one if you need discretion. Here is CARINA's suggestion for a "total facial experience" for all ages:

- *"Personalised aromatherapy as chosen by your consultant and led by your nose*
- *Skin analysis by touch*
- *Hot cotton towel hand mitts with suitable essential oils added to soften the water and create a wonderful Aroma*
- *Facial massage with lymphatic drainage*
- *Deeply relaxing massage with acupressure*
- *Pre-heated Purifying or Revitalising Urban Sense Clay Mask*
- *Specialised and experienced deep massage to the face, neck, shoulders and scalp*
- *Foot Spa with Marine salt crystals and olive leaf oil from Planet Botanic*
- *Unique ice massage over dampened gauze for 30–60 seconds to stimulate and revitalise and cool the skin*
- *Foot and arm experience with hot towels with chosen essential oils and body/foot butters from Est*
- *Soothing mask using simply pure Aloe Vera*
- *Abdomen massage with pre-heated prescribed blend to aid digestion and release tension*
- *Finish with a foot massage with cocoa butter."*

CARINA COEN

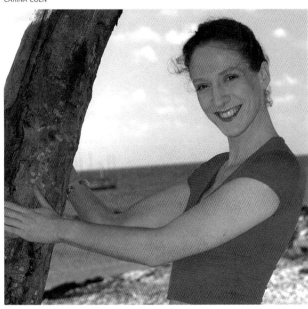

HOME BEAUTY TREATMENTS

from Sidra Shaukat

For those of us who do not have huge budgets to spend on our beauty regimes, the answer is home treatments using every day domestic ingredients. Here is an excerpt from beauty expert SIDRA SHAUKAT's highly practical book, *Natural Beauty*:

It's very tempting to buy the most expensive cream with its promises of eternal youth and expect to look years younger. However, the majority of women are very disappointed when there is no significant change in their looks. These creams are little more than expensive moisturisers.

There is a way, however, to look your very best using natural treatments with ingredients from your kitchen. Taken from my international bestseller, *Natural Beauty*, (visit www.sidrashaukat.biz for details) these treatments are simple, effective and economical.

Exfoliating

Exfoliation, however executed, speeds up the rate of cell renewal and is essential as you get older because the metabolism slows down. Exfoliate, to dislodge dead skin cells, by performing brisk brush ups with a loofah or massage mitt which will get skin glowing. Or use finely ground oatmeal, a good gentle exfoliator, which makes an effective scrub before a shower. Simply rub all over. For a cheap face scrub and good exfoliator, mix a small amount of sugar (preferably coarse such as granulated sugar) with your favourite cleanser. Massage over your face and wash off thoroughly. This acts in the same way as the expensive gels with exfoliating "beads" in them, but is also gentler and much cheaper.

Steaming

Steam unclogs pores to deep cleanse skin and soften it. Use a deep bowl and fill with boiling water. Immerse face towards steam and cover head with a towel around edges of the bowl to prevent steam escaping.

The steam will penetrate and open the pores to bring the dirt to the surface. Tone with a non-alcoholic toner applied with cotton wool to close and tighten pores. Repeat weekly.

Tea acts as a mild tonic and conditioner, so a steaming tea facial will deep cleanse the skin. Pour hand hot tea into a bowl or sink, add a few dashes of lemon rind and some marjoram and mint (dried type will do). Now lean your face over the bowl and head with towel. The heat and toning polyphenols in the tea will draw out impurities.

Face masks

All skins benefit from a face mask which deep cleanses and refines. For dry skin, try an avocado night mask. Mash a ripe avocado into a cream or liquidise, smooth onto face and relax for 15 minutes. Tissue away most of the cream but leave a trace on the skin's surface. During the night, the remaining oils will condition and soften the skin.

To treat the odd blemish, dip a cotton bud in witch hazel and dab directly onto area. At bedtime, soak a cotton wool ball in calamine lotion and apply directly onto area.

Lemon juice is a well known cure for sallow oily skin, which makes it an ideal ingredient in face masks etc. Lemon juice is good for spot-prone skin because it neutralises bacteria and contains high levels of Vitamin C to heal the skin. Rub a slice of lemon over skin and rinse with cold water.

A clean face flannel dipped in hot water placed on the face while lying down, is an instant relaxer. To freshen or revive a tired face, dip clean flannel in ice-cold water and place on face for five minutes. Your face will have a healthy pinky glow, signifying increased blood circulation to the surface of the skin. Your eyes will sparkle too, as all the puffiness will be eliminated.

Make several skin fresheners with cucumber, which is good for normal skins, especially oily to combination skins. Puree a few slices of peeled cucumber (or you can

grate them if it is easier and quicker) with two tablespoons of natural yoghurt. Use as a face mask for half an hour and rinse off with lukewarm water.

Create your own spa at home

Spas are no longer the preserve of the rich and famous, now that they are within the price range of everyday folk. They have increased in popularity due to special deals, and highly stressful lives making them a necessity rather than a luxury. I often create my own spa at home using my natural treatments.

You may want to invite your best friend over for some of the body treatments, and take it in turns to pamper each other. Most of the ingredients can be purchased over the counter at larger chemists.

1 Face and body mask

When we think of a spa, the first thing we think of is the face and body covered with a green mud mask. Mud is fantastic for drawing out impurities from the skin to leave it glowing. A shower afterwards, as cold as you can bear, does wonders for the circulation.

I make a green clay and turmeric mask (turmeric is the yellow spice used in curries that is a great cleanser) by mixing one heaped tablespoon of green clay with one teaspoon of turmeric and mixing in live yoghurt or water if you prefer to make it a thick paste. If you have dry skin, you may want to add a little almond oil as required. This is enough for the face, make larger amounts for the body. You can obtain my mask to order (sent same day) online at www.sidrashaukat.biz.

For oily skins, make a clay mask by mixing one whisked egg white with one tablespoon of Fuller's Earth (from chemists). Add a few drops of peppermint oil. Leave to dry and rinse with lukewarm water.

For dry skins, whisk one egg white; mix with one teaspoon of honey. Put on with a pastry brush and leave for ten minutes. Wash off with cold water. The egg white gives this mask its firming effect.

2 Baths

Your bath could be the equivalent of the spa bath for its treatment properties. Cleopatra bathed in ass's milk to maintain her beauty, you can do the same too! Instead of ass's milk, you can add ¼ pint of milk to the running water, or try two tablespoons of dried milk for the same effect. For added indulgence, a few drops of coconut essence will give the bath a tropical feel.

You can even create the effect of being in a thermal mud bath known for its therapeutic effects by just adding two or three tablespoons of green clay or Fuller's Earth to the running warm water.

Sink into a warm bath scented with essential oils such as ylang-ylang, patchouli or rosemary (to clear the head) and lavender, rose or camomile (to relax and soothe). Make sure the water is not too hot, as this over stimulates the nervous system and reduces the oils' therapeutic powers. To make this indulgent soak extra special, put on some soft, soothing music, dim the lights in the bathroom and relax.

Bathing is an excellent way of relaxing after a hard day, but over using commercial bath preparations can dry out your skin. Herbal baths are a refreshing alternative and are useful for cystitis sufferers who should avoid perfumed bubble baths and oils.

Tie a handful of fresh herbs in some muslin and place in the bath under the taps. Run the hot water first to release the scent from the herbs, and then top up with cold water. Try lovage, camomile (you could even use camomile teabags or herbal teabags!), mint or rosemary. Out of season, you can use dried herbs instead of fresh herbs. A drop of baby oil, wheat germ oil or almond oil will stop your skin from drying out.

3 Face and body scrubs and exfoliators

There are various sea salt scrubs available on the market, but you can make your own or buy my special recipe sea salt scrub with coconut oil and lavender at www.sidrashaukat.biz/scrub.

Raw sea salt is available from most supermarkets. Just mix with your favourite body oil, coconut oil being the best and rub vigorously all over the body. If you have sensitive skin, use granulated sugar instead of salt. Pay particular attention to the thighs to reduce and prevent cellulite.

Face scrubs will clear and brighten the complexion. Try a peach face scrub. Mash a large ripe peach, or liquidise using a food processor, mix with a dessertspoon of oatmeal and rub all over the face. Rinse with warm water.

Try a nutty facial scrub for soft skin. Crush 4 oz blanched almonds to a fine paste. Add one egg and two teaspoons of rose water. Mix well. Using your fingertips, rub the mixture gently into the oily areas of your face and leave for ten minutes before rinsing off well.

Grape juice is an effective natural exfoliator, removing dead skin cells and brightening the skin. Grape seed oil is also a good, light moisturiser for normal to dry skin. Apples too are natural skin exfoliators; just cut a slice and whisk it over your face.

4 Hair removal

You may want to purchase wax and use it at home. I have created an extra special wax which is totally natural, made from just lemon juice, sugar, beeswax and honey. You can get your hands on some at www.sidrashaukat.biz/wax. Or if you are feeling adventurous, try making your own.

In the Middle East, it is customary for the bride to be removed of all body hair. This is done using only natural products such as water, sugar, lemon juice and honey. One method is sugaring, which consists of purely water and sugar, heated gently, in different combinations, depending on the preference of the user.

Sugaring can be tricky to perfect but the time spent on practising can save time, money and the results are smooth, stubble-free skin which will remain hair-free for up to eight weeks.

Try the one to one technique to start off with, using one tablespoon of water to one tablespoon of granulated sugar, in a metal

pan, over gentle heat. When the sugar dissolves, and the liquid is the consistency of honey, allow it to cool slightly, and when at body temperature, spoon on mixture with a metal spoon or spatula.

Press mixture onto skin with hands or use a strip of cotton to press mixture against the skin. Pull off mixture with hands or take off strip against hair growth. Rinse with cold water.

You will notice a lovely sheen on the skin. You can vary combinations of sugar to water depending on how thick you like the mixture, and the consistency you find easiest to work with.

Once you are familiar with the technique, you can make larger amounts in the same proportions of sugar to water. You may find it messy at first, but after practice, it will be fuss and mess free!

Hair treatments

Treat **over-dry hair** and scalp to a pre-shampoo oil pack. Gently heat olive, almond or jojoba oil in a saucer over a pan of boiling water, apply to dry hair and massage in well. Wrap your head in foil or an old towel and sit in the bath for 15 minutes (the steam will help the oil penetrate your hair and scalp). To wash the oil out, apply shampoo directly to the hair without rinsing first, massage, and rinse and then shampoo again as normal.

To smooth and brighten **dull hair**, beat an egg yolk, add to a small carton of yoghurt and beat thoroughly. Shampoo hair then comb the yoghurt and egg mixture through it. Leave on for 10–15 minutes, then rinse thoroughly with lukewarm water.

Prevent **split ends** by working mayonnaise into clean dry hair and leaving it on for at least an hour. Use either the purer commercial mayonnaise without harmful additives or simply make your own by whisking one teaspoon each of oil (vegetable, sunflower or almond) and vinegar along with one large egg, until well blended and glossy in appearance.

Hair rinse To prevent dandruff, and give your hair a fresh perfume, try a rosemary hair rinse. Put a large handful of rosemary into a pan and cover with water. Simmer for 10–15 minutes, then leave to cool. Strain the mixture using a sieve into a jug containing a few drops of wheat germ oil or any oil.

Use as an after-shampoo rinse, washing hair first with a very mild shampoo. Finally rinse thoroughly with tepid water.

For **natural hair colouring**, try herbal rinses to give a soft, subtle effect. Camomile flowers add sheen to blonde hair, nettles are a good tonic for all hair types, but be careful gathering them, and elderberries will add a subtle deep mahogany colour to dark hair. Put a large handful of the appropriate plant

into a pan and cover completely with water. Simmer for 20 minutes, strain and leave to cool. After washing hair with a mild shampoo, use the rinse. Rinse thoroughly with cool water, ensuring that no rinse remains.

Hair removal

Then there is the prickly problem of when to start plucking and waxing, remembering that this is for life, girls! My advice is to leave your legs and bikini area as long as possible: fine hair gets bleached in the sun and teenagers can get away with it. The eyebrows are a different matter: the brows define the eyes and as soon as young girls start wearing make-up they want to attend to their brows. It is very important to go to a reputable salon when you first start plucking and waxing: young skin is easily scarred and you can ruin the line of your brows for life if you over pluck. Ask the beautician to show you how to pluck properly and do not "have a go" yourself until you know exactly what you are doing! The same goes for waxing which is even trickier to do at home. This is what VANESSA of VANESSA'S HAIR AND BEAUTY (201 North End Road, West Kensington, W14 9NL, phone 020 7385 3674) who specialises in treating young customers has to say:

"Eyebrows are extremely important. They can make a person look anxious, happy, sad, angry, surprised or confused. They are an expression of the face that we recognise in our early teenage years and we need advice on their shape and daily grooming. The best advice is to keep their natural shape and to frame the eyes without overwhelming them and to pluck only in order to enhance what you have naturally.

VANESSA ANN GILLIES

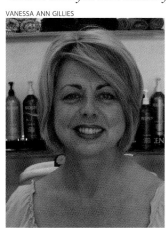

A qualified beautician that you can trust will advise you on the best natural shape for your face and show you how to maintain them in between visits to the salon. Reshaping is necessary in some cases due to eyebrows being overgrown. A good tip: very thin eyebrows can age you and to make them look bushy or thicker pencil them in or have a professional eye brow tint applied."

There are so many different hair and beauty treatments available now; which are the best for you personally? HAIR AND BEAUTY VARIATIONS, the posh but reasonable salon at FORTNUM AND MASON owned by NEIL WARD (181 Piccadilly, W1A 1ER, phone 020 7437 3424) reports:

"Facials are our most popular beauty treatments, especially the 'Caviar Treatments' using the expensive but superior LA PRAIRIE range of products. Our beauticians find that the quality of the LA PRAIRIE creams is the very best which is important because a good facial relies on the quality of the products used as well as the facial massage.

Our BOWEN massage technique has proved very successful for body treatments; it is a soft touch massage that really gets to the areas that need relaxing".

HBV recently acquired an amazing new machine called the GENIE COMPLETE which seems in my humble opinion to be By Royal Appointment. Read on:

"When CAMILLA (THE DUCHESS OF CORNWALL) was preparing for her wedding she wanted to look svelte and to achieve this, she had a series of treatments using the Ultimate Slimming and Toning System, the GENIE COMPLETE, otherwise known as a personal trainer for the face and the body. HBV is one of the few salons to offer this wonderful selection of treatments. This brilliant system's most attractive feature is that it is ultra speedy, sometimes only ten minutes are required. (DR RONALD BAXENDALE invented the ten-minute face-lift which uses safe 'waves' that are a thousand times stronger than anything else available, so that it only takes ten minutes to get visible results.)

The GENIE can also be used for a power body tone that takes a mere twenty minutes to help with cellulite, loose skin, stretch marks and bust lifting. GENIE COMPLETE is also good for lymphatic drainage, which again encourages rapid inch loss and detoxing of the lymph. There is also a Diamond Eyes Treatment which helps lift droopy eyelids. In short, THE GENIE is a miraculous system – what better way to spend lunchtime?"

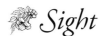

Now here is the hair news from HAIR AND BEAUTY VARIATIONS. *"We have the only long hair clinic in London for ladies with naturally long locks (not extensions) and it is very popular. We also find that many ladies are taking advantage of our stylists who specialise in 'up do's' to achieve a more elegant look, especially for evenings. Our bridal service is also doing very well; brides and their entourages always like to be pampered for 'the big day'."*

Hair colour and styling

Ladies often like to have a complete make over of their hairstyle and our guest stylist and colourist PATRICK LUDDE offers this service. PATRICK specialises in the subtle colour that makes older ladies look younger and young ones look modern. He takes great care with products so as not to overload the hair: "fragile hair is ugly hair", he believes. PATRICK spends much of his time working with the world's top models and photographers and he will make *you* look like a top model!

I talked to PAOLO SANNA, the manager of HAIR AND BEAUTY VARIATIONS who is also a film and TV hair stylist and colouring expert. PAOLO said: *"When you want to colour your hair you must also discuss the style with your colourist. For blondes I like to use as little bleach as possible as it damages the hair and makes it very dry. Luckily the fashion today is for warmer blonde tones which can be achieved with a high lifting tint rather than the brassy look you get with bleach. I see a lot of problems today with hair loss and damaged hair due to over processing or the use of bleach so I always try to use more natural products.*

For highlights I always use foil or 'Easy Meche' which are much better for the hair than the cap system. I only use the cap for hair which is too short to wrap.

Red is the hardest colour to achieve; you should always do a test first. You can use henna to redden the hair naturally but it does not last very long and you will need to use a tint to create a permanent redhead.

Brunette tones are the easiest to achieve and are used a lot for covering grey hair. Black-black is not popular any more but blue-black and violet-black look great on young people.

Cutting is all important to create good styles. Natural (i.e. without extensions) long hair needs a lot of maintenance and you must condition it regularly. The secret of a good conditioning product is in the PH balance; the same can be said for anti dandruff products.

Blow drying is best for straight hair styles but soft, wavy styles are coming back now and they require a good set on rollers. Heated rollers and tongs are very damaging for the hair as, unlike hot air drying, they actually touch the hair and can burn it so try not to use them if you can avoid it.

I always hate it when a client says to me 'I want to look like so and so' (usually some film star or other) because they may not have the right physical appearance for that style. Sometimes you have to compromise to suit your own particular look or style. But then you are unique, not just a shadow of someone else."

PAOLO's advice about heated rollers and tongs is extremely valuable: sometimes you can actually hear your poor hair sizzling! Do not even think about crimping or ironing your locks: these gadgets are for waffles and materials, not for hair. Although Hollywood film producer extraordinaire PATRICK CURTIS says he used to regularly iron his gorgeous former wife RAQUEL WELCH's lustrous locks, I would say this is *not* something to try at home!

Hair extensions

Hair extensions have become a fact of life now and ladies are using this amazing modern technique to gain thickness as well as length. Celebrity salon owner JANET GINNINGS (JANET GINNINGS SALON 45 Curzon Street, Mayfair, W1, phone 020 7499 2767, www.janetginnings.co.uk) looks after the hair and skin of numerous high profile beauties including supermodels ELLE MCPHERSON and CAPRICE, TV gals KATY HILL and MEERA SYAL, PR guru LIZ BREWER and LIZ's high flying client IVANA TRUMP.

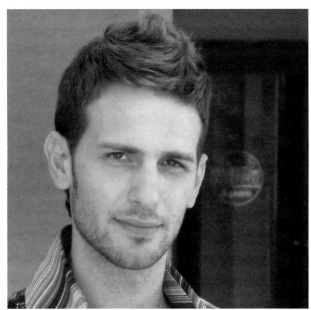

PAOLO SANNA

One of Janet's favourite extensions clients CAPRICE reckons *"JANET's are simply the best extensions in the world"*. JANET told me: *"Hair extensions come in a variety of different systems and you can now choose from monofibre synthetic materials or real hair extensions that are attached at the root for an extra natural look. Extensions take about three hours to put in and last approximately three months. After three months you remove them and put fresh ones in. You can have all sorts of different colours, for instance to achieve a highlighted look without colouring your own hair."*

Non-surgical face lift

THE JANET GINNINGS SALON also offers all the usual beauty treatments as well as hairdos and boasts the fastest hair setter in town, ALZIRA DE FREITAS. VIP clients can book JANET herself who is an amazing hair cutter, stylist and beauty therapist. Celeb socialite MEG MATTHEWS favours JANET's RIGENERA regenerating facial. She says *"JANET has magical hands: I had the best facial I have ever had. I cannot believe this treatment was under my nose the whole time. People have been commenting on how fab my skin looks"*. JANET says: *"Facials are fast becoming a beauty necessity largely due to the stress and strain of everyday life which leaves tell tale lines on our faces. It is imperative to hold back the hands of time with regular facials that will ensure your face is left looking vibrant, supple and youthful. Our latest RIGENERA facial, known as 'the non surgical face lift' or 'face gym', which MEG likes so much is brilliant. The therapist will manually 'work out' all the individual facial muscles, including the all important eye area, with specific hand movements to gently lift the face, restore skin tone and elasticity and smooth out wrinkles. The procedure really improves circulation and oxygenation and accelerates tissue regeneration.*

With technology that is second to none we are now also able to offer our clients the famous OXYJET anti-ageing facial which actually uses pure oxygen to give the skin a healthy glow and ensure that it looks fresh and youthful at all times. CAPRICE, for instance, is very keen on the OXYJET facial."

Waxing

You can also keep up with the latest waxing trend at JANET's salon, the BOLLYWOOD wax. The BOLLYWOOD is one step up from the BRAZILIAN inasmuch as it leaves you totally smooth downstairs and adorned with SWAROVSKI crystals: just the job if you want to be a sexy goddess and make your guy sit up and take notice!

Nails

Do not forget to include regular manicures and pedicures in your beauty regime: people really do notice the extremities and it is important to achieve a totally groomed look. JANET says: *"The technology behind manicures and pedicures is advancing at great speed and there are now literally hundreds of different*

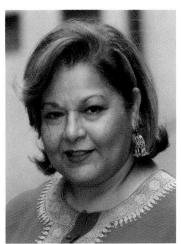

JANET GINNINGS

nail systems to choose from. If you are a lady who likes to be pampered, take the time to have it done properly with our 'Indian Kitchen Manicure and Pedicure' where rose petals and goat's milk are used for the ultimate luxury."

If your nails are weak and just will not grow however much MAVALA and SALLY HANSEN you use you may need to have them sculptured. Whether you go for silk wraps (which have a thinner, more delicate appearance), gel (slightly safer than acrylic) or acrylic itself, it is vital to go to a really good salon to protect your nail health. TYRONE AND COMPANY (14 Porchester Place, Marble Arch, W2 2BF, phone 020 7723 4843, www.tyroneandcompany.com) is an excellent salon awash with celebs where you really can be beautified "from top to toe". TYRONE has an excellent nail technician called LEONE who also specialises in Nail Art to decorate the nails once they are long and gorgeous.

If you prefer your nail technician to come to you

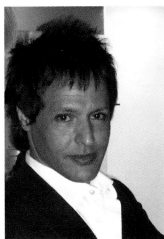

TYRONE

CLARE SMITH (07957 60 59 63) is excellent and will travel to anywhere within London and the Home Counties. CLARE says *"You should have your sculptured nails 'filled in' every three to four weeks. I use a holistic UB gel which is non-acrylic and non harmful. It is the only nail enhancement product that I use and it is independently clinically tested. You must be careful* where you go to get your nails done and do not go to a salon where they use machines as these can damage the nail plate or even the nail bed."

Getting back to the TYRONE salon, TYRONE himself is a TV and media hair and make-up artiste who is absolutely superb at creating big hair styles, both up and down. As we big haired ladies say, "size matters"! Here TYRONE tells us why he agrees with us:

"Yes! Big Hair is back for the noughties! With the colour techniques used today coupled with superb hair products, Big Hair can look more amazing than ever.

Sensational looks are what people want today and to be extrovert in ones appearance seems to be totally acceptable – and for all ages. A glamorous gown can be crowned with a mane of voluminous hair, coloured to perfection and conditioned to give maximum shine. A head turner for that dramatic entrance! Or beautifully sculpted hair with a quiff to set off that tailored suit. Big, Bold and Beautiful is my motto for the look of today."

For those of you London dwellers or visitors who are women on the move, now you can be beautified from top to toe all at once. Brand new salon MONOCHROME Body And Soul (38–39 Duke of York's Square, King's Road, London, SW3 4LY, phone 020 7602 6253) can do your hair, facial, waxing, manicure and pedicure all together: brilliant.

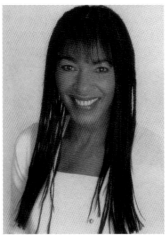
EVA LEWIS

MONOCHROME, owned by showbiz entrepreneur EVA LEWIS is the first salon to look after all skin colours and types of hair as well as being unisex (they do have private treatment rooms of course!) It is also the first British salon I have found to offer the excellent CARITA treatments beloved of beauty expert NORMANDIE KEITH, including their latest lifting innovation for the face, PRO-LIFT.

This salon is very well laid out with a social area offering food and drink, a nail bar, showers for before and after tanning and vibrating chairs. Check it out.

Wigs

On the hair front if you suffer from serious hair loss which cannot be helped with trichology treatments from the top salons, try REGAINE FOR WOMEN (020 7815 3900 or e-mail firstname.secondname@munroforster.com). REGAINE, you may remember, is the scalp solution which MICHAEL WINNER famously used to maintain his leonine silver mane. A HOT GOSSIP UK "Product of the Month", REGAINE works just as well for women and will not just prevent further hair loss but actually regrow hair. Its active ingredient is Minoxidil which has been clinically proven to be effective in treating hair loss and it works by stimulating the hair follicles to encourage growth. It is every woman's right to have "full-on gorgeous hair" so fight for it, ladies.

While your hair is growing, or maybe just for fun or to try a colour change, check out the wig scene. TRENDCO (020 7221 2646, www.trendcowigs.co.uk) is the biggest name in the UK for both real hair and acrylic wigs and hairpieces. Their "wigglies" and "ferrets" as I fondly call these hair accessories can be either very natural looking or frankly fake. They can be lots of fun especially if you are having a bad hair day, but please note the shocking pink and purple jobbies to match your frox are strictly fancy dress time!

Spas

If you really want to pamper yourself and maybe need to lose a bit of weight and/or stop smoking or drinking in congenial surroundings amongst like minded ladies (and some gentlemen!) a health farm is the answer. There is no shortage of wonderful hydros, or "fat farms" as the skinny Lizzies like to call them, in the UK including GRAYSHOTT, FOREST MERE, HENLOW GRANGE, CHAMPNEYS, RAGDALE HALL, SHRUBLANDS, et al. The range of treatments available at these luxurious establishments is mind blowing but anything with seaweed in will be both slimming and detoxing. As CAZ PETT, spa manager at the popular and showbizzy FOREST MERE, says *"algae contains relatively high levels of iodine which speed up the metabolism".*

Medispa treatments

MEDISPA is a spa with a difference. Not only does it offer all the usual treatments but it boasts its own cosmetic doctor, DR ROY SALEH, MBChB, who can give you a Medispa Midface Lipo Lift during your stay. Read on for details of MEDISPA and the MFLL:

MEDISPA AND THE MFLL

from Dr Roy Saleh

The utter delight and benefit of "letting" go in a Spa should never be underestimated by any budding health goddess. Many women go feeling like a dull, dying moth and embrace the cocooning escape a good Spa will bring.

Spas, like people, come in different sizes and pleasures and perhaps the most unique are the popular Medispa clinics which offer under one roof all the sensual pleasures from pampering, massage and delicious aroma oils to stringent detox, salt scrubs and G5 pummelling guaranteed to "break" up the most stubborn fat.

Many ladies say the benefits of the above treatments make them feel as if they are shedding a skin. To finish off the bliss of a face and scalp massage combined with an ozone steam helps create a tunnel of recovery and the gentle tweaking and manipulation during massage of the eyebrow can diminish the most ferocious of headaches and tensions and increase "endorphins", the body's natural antibiotic to stress, to create a wellness and feel good factor.

As well as experiencing the beauty side, you can request a "rejuvenation" session to aid facial enhancement. Over the last 25 years I have put up an aesthetic umbrella to prevent ladies from ageing further, thus preserving and discreetly enhancing their facial appearance.

I spend 35–45 minutes "face mapping" each client to help me understand "her individual" way of ageing and to help me prepare a 12-month rejuvenation strategy and then simple maintenance programmes afterwards. The art of combining beauty alongside non-surgical treatments such as Botox, fillers and volumising is an incredibly effective and clever "preventative tool" as one approaches different "stages" in life to preserve and perhaps enhance one's appearance. It helps to take away the stress of worrying about having to resort to surgery and having a constantly "tired look" even on the happiest of occasions.

It has often been said that at 40 you have to choose between your face or your figure – now you can have both! – the Medispa way.

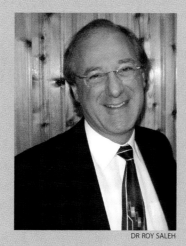

DR ROY SALEH

From my youth I have always had a passion for photographing faces. Balancing the proportion and symmetry of the face has always intrigued me and the effect of "unattractiveness" and the different ways it can be perceived.

I realised that the better people looked the better they felt about themselves. If you look in the mirror and what you see pleases you it gives you enormous confidence and on occasions happiness.

When I became a doctor I worked in Accident and Emergency and was always given the treatments which involved the repair of facial lacerations. I spent such a lot of time on it. The repair of the human face became my vocation – the better the job I did on a patient's face the better they would be able to live with their scars.

Years later when I became involved in facial screening in relation to cosmetic facial surgery, I became interested and curious as to why people wanted cosmetic surgery – what happened to the ones that were not suitable or ready for facial surgery? At that point I realised that cosmetic surgery should be considered as a last resort.

So I researched and developed expertise and knowledge in all the procedures that didn't involve cosmetic surgery. I was fortunate to have good teachers and I soon realised that I could prevent or slow down the need for many procedures that would have been traditionally done by surgery

such as eyelid, brow, face and veins.

Over the last 35 years my passion and dedication for non-surgical facial enhancement have grown. It has become my life. I have continued to develop my expertise and knowledge on a daily full time basis and have been able to pioneer and introduce new facial aesthetic techniques and procedures into people's everyday lives.

The Medispa Midface lipo lift (MFLL) In the late 1980s I had been injecting collagen which was relatively expensive and I had a client who was unsuitable for facial surgery but suitable for non surgical enhancement. Sadly she told me she could no longer afford to continue with collagen so I offered to remove her fat and inject it into her face to replace the collagen injection. This was immensely successful and the client was delighted.

At the same time I also had a patient referred to me who was suitable for a face lift but her husband was against the operation and its risks. After a consultation I was able to recommend a MFLL which would give her the same result as a face lift without the risk – no surgery or general anaesthetic. Both were delighted by the treatment. The husband was not worried; the wife he loved was not to be operated on, in bandages or hospitalised. However she was able to see a pleasing improvement and felt that her procedure was worth while.

MFLL Procedure This is a medical procedure designed and performed exclusively by me. The whole process takes approximately three hours and can be split into two parts for the convenience and care of the patient. It does not involve hospitalisation and allays any fear of operations and anaesthetic.

All patients are examined personally to ascertain suitability.

MFLL Stage 1

- Removal of fat from the body
- Injection of fat into the face
- Fat can be removed from any where in the body but the preferred areas are the abdomen and hips
- The fat is very gently extracted from an area measuring 4 × 4 inches. This is a highly skilled procedure, as it is crucial to

ensure that the fat is removed evenly and great care is taken not to damage the fat.

This part of the procedure involves injecting a local anaesthetic under the skin in an area of about the size of the hand.

Once the area is anaesthetised, a needle is attached to a syringe and the fat is syringed out through a tiny hole. This is a gentle, painless procedure unlike liposuction. Again it is essential not to damage the fat. This process takes approximately one and a half hours.

A bandage is applied to the area and a support garment is supplied and should be worn for at least a week.

The fat is cleaned and stored in syringes and then deep frozen. Each syringe is numbered and labelled and coded: date of extraction, patient's DOB and identification number. It is then put in its own individual container, stored in a special freezer. The fat is never removed from deep freeze until the patient arrives at the clinic.

Associated risks

- Discomfort for a few days
- Leakage of stained fluid through tiny hole overnight
- Bruising and possible contour irregularities.

MFLL Stage 2

The re injection of fat into the face takes 1½ hours.

This process can be done immediately afterwards or on a separate occasion. I mark the facial areas that require augmentation/enhancement. These marked areas are injected with local anaesthetic – (similar to going to a dentist).

Small needle holes are discreetly made near the ear and jaw line to avoid marks and bruising on the main part of the face.

The procedure fills the face to make you look eight years younger.

The little needle holes are sealed with steri strip and a protective mask is applied, which gently supports the face and reduces swelling and bruising.

This is a procedure without the frightening risks of surgery. It is designed to fill and give youthful volume to the face and has the result of enabling patients to look eight years younger and to easily maintain that look throughout their life. Normally done twice during the first year, then every year to replenish and maintain.

I have designed this treatment to ensure the enhancement effect gets better each

year, due to the yearly replenishing and building of the fat.

Is face lifting my only option?

From the minute you do a face lift you are deteriorating – If you are replenishing the padding of the face once a year you do not deteriorate.

If you lose facial padding (fat) your face drops – when people get old, the fat goes (fat atrophy) and the skin drops.

Up till now no one has really thought about the importance of fat and the part it plays in maintaining youthfulness.

The focus has been on surgery – to cut. Modern surgery pulls the muscle and skin up – but doesn't replace the padding surgically hence the face looks tighter and on some occasions hollowed but not fuller. Instead the padding (fat) gives a person a youthfulness, a sensual roundness and symmetry, which is pleasing.

The MFLL is a non- surgical treatment which gives our Medispa clients a face lift appearance but without surgery or any scars and the comfort that they can maintain and enhance their looks every year for the rest of their lives.

Cosmetic surgeon MR EDWARD LATIMER-SAYER, BSc MB BS FRCS (01590 623226, a/p/s: 020 8731 7021, www.latimer-sayer.co.uk) also advocates the "autologous fat transfer" which he uses in conjunction with a face lift to counteract any hollowness. MR LATIMER-SAYER is of course the surgeon who transformed cosmetic surgery guru CINDY JACKSON (020 8340 0205, www.cindyjackson.com) from a plain Idaho farm girl into the beauteous lady who looks "more like BARBIE than BARBIE". He is also a fan of dermabrasion, either on its own or with a face lift, which he says has the same effect as a chemical peel or laser but is not so painful. I will deal with cosmetic surgery and serious cosmetic procedures in a later chapter where we will be hearing from CINDY JACKSON, EDWARD LATIMER-SAYER and other famous cosmetic surgeons.

More spas

Getting back to spas, health and beauty lovers, I suggest you choose spa or "resort" hotels when you go on holiday. For instance I chose the world renowned LE SPORT HOTEL in ST LUCIA (001 758 450 8551) for my honeymoon with my sporty husband JEREMY; it is just so relaxing for your mind and body to finish off an energetic day of scuba diving or water skiing with a bit of pampering.

The KEMPINSKI INTERNATIONAL (020 8307 7657) hotels are amongst the most luxurious in the world and include eleven "resort hotels" where you can indulge in all your favourite beauty treatments as well as enjoying the sporting activities on offer and eating five star food. For instance the fabulously pretty KEMPINSKI, ESTEPONA (0034 952 809500) on the main MARBELLA drag includes the POLLYMAR spa with treatments by POLLY HILLBRUNNER, the lady who invented the body wrap.

The KEMPINSKI, SAN LAWRENZ (0035 622 110000) on the picturesque baby island of GOZO is my personal favourite for summer holidays and not just because you can bump into BRAD PITT and SEAN CONNERY there! Apart from using the gym, playing tennis, swimming in three pools and eating in three restaurants you can try all the amazing treatments in the hotel's world famous AYURVEDA CENTRE, beloved of the UK's legendary diarist NIGEL DEMPSTER. You can have all the usual treatments such as facials, massages, manicures and pedicures and try a spot of the Ayurvedic technique as well, including an extraordinary treatment where the therapist massages you while hanging from a rope! My particular favourite is the Indian Head Massage (leave the oil in overnight and wash your hair in the morning: you will have to wear your hair in a tight knot or a bandanna that evening but it will be worth it).

One of the most divine KEMPINSKI hotels is the ST MORITZ one which is a year round resort with some of the best skiing (and night life) in the world in winter and the delights of alpine rambling, not to mention R and R, in the summer when there is usually more time to "take the waters". To my mind the KSM offers the perfect healthy winter holiday; the combination of being able to ski all day and take the waters, cleanse your skin in the sauna and enjoy pampering treatments in the well equipped spa before dinner is my idea of Heaven (or at least a health goddess's Heaven!) The beauty treatments and spa facilities at

CINDY JACKSON

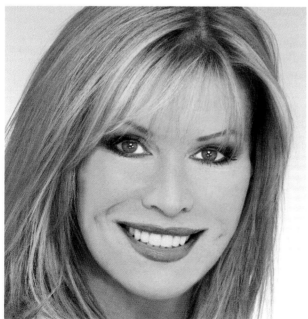

the KEMPINSKI GRAND HOTEL DES BAINS (7500 St Moritz, Switzerland, phone 0041 81 838 3838, e-mail reservations.grandhoteldesbains@kempinski.com) are second to none and there is a medical spa nearby where you can have diagnosis and treatment from a wide range of doctors. The KSM's charming manager MR RUPERT SIMONER says:

"We are the only authentic Alpine Spa and work closely with local farmers and universities who produce our ingredients. Our philosophy is to use local alpine resources and re-discover the strengths which were known over centuries but have been forgotten. On the beauty side we are the only hotel Spa worldwide which works directly with Valmont (a very exclusive Swiss based brand) which incorporates only local produce, glacier water and DNS structure cosmetics into their products.

The design of the entire Spa area is alpine too – but contemporary. Sleek granite stone walls, dark wood, open spaces, cosy corners and definitely no 'Kitsch' as we say… The 'birthplace' of St Moritz is within the Spa – the Mauritius source which is accessible for hotel residents. Its healing waters were discovered by Paracelsus and made St Moritz famous. The Spa is built around it.

The Spa concept has been named already in its first year one of the top 3 Spas in Switzerland and amongst the top ten in Europe."

Several hotels in London now have fitness centres and spas and I am delighted to report that my favourite London hotel, THE DORCHESTER has recently revamped its beautiful Spa which is now managed by ANN COSTELLOE. "Ladies who Dorch" can still have all the usual beauty treatments, get their hair done in the worthy CHARLES WORTHINGTON salon and have champagne tea after working out in the State of the Art gymnasium. However the Spa now also offers a brilliant new treatment called "The Bi-Aura Stress Buster" where qualified practitioner DAN KAHN will work on your personal stress. The "Stress Buster" works on and penetrates into the areas of the body affected by stress, returning the energy flow to normal, clearing blockages and allowing the body and mind to enter into a deep state of relaxation. So visitors to our delightful capital can now keep fit, healthy and stress free as well as being deliciously and nutritiously fed whilst staying at the famous DORCHESTER.

Sight

13

THE SUN & ITS EFFECTS

& FAKE TANS

It would be impossible to write a health and beauty book without mentioning the damaging and ageing effects of the sun. Lying in the sun is extremely sensually pleasurable, especially after a long, hard British winter. Although some gentle sun exposure is good for our flora and fauna and makes us feel good, its intense rays are extremely bad for your health and looks; skin cancer can kill you and exposure to the sun will dry and age your skin, much more than any of the other elements. If I had known in my tender youth what I now, in middle age, know about the sun, I would never have cooked myself for years, ending up with sun damaged skin.

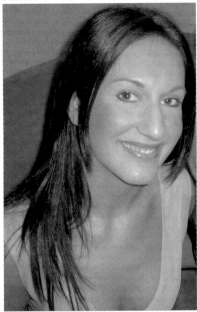

LAURA FERRALL-PEEVEY

You simply must protect your skin from the sun by wearing hats, staying in the shade at midday and using a good sun cream with an SPF of 30 or higher or indeed a total sun block. No ifs or buts: the only ladies I know with really good skin are those who have always protected themselves from those naughty rays. You may be able to laser or microdermabrade your facial skin or indeed try other more radical treatments or surgery which we will discuss in later chapters on your face. However, it is impossible to treat your whole body and limbs. So please take my advice and stay in the shade as much as possible and wear a very high SPF when you do have to be in the sun, for example if you are into water sports. Also try to keep out of the sun during the hottest part of the day, which is, after all, the ideal time for a long, leisurely (and healthy!) lunch anyway.

It is never too late to start protecting yourself from the sun but prevention is better than cure so, if you are young, get into the habit of using sun protection creams at all times, especially in the summer. If you have children please do them a favour and do the same for their delicate skins. Luckily there are loads of wonderful sun protection products on the market nowadays. All the top cosmetics and skin care manufacturers have a range of sun care products so there is no excuse for getting caught out looking like a lobster ever again. If you live in a sunny climate you will probably get a light colour from just walking around, even if you use a high SPF and try to stay in the shade but you must avoid actually getting burnt at all costs.

Products

I tend to use LANCÔME facial products in the summer because their "Soleil Soft-Touch Effect" Anti Wrinkle Cream and Moisturising Lotion have a high SPF and I use their sun care products as well, especially on my

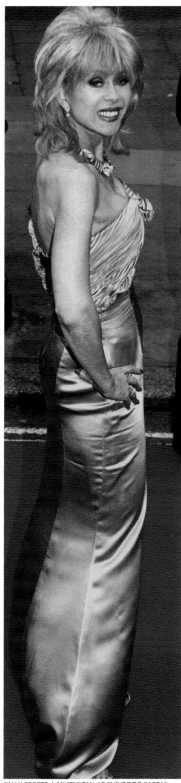

SALLY SPORTS A MYSTIC TAN AT THE 2005 BAFTAS
DRESS BY ROUBI EL ROUBI
PHOTO: ROWENA CHOWDREY

face and lips. The LANCÔME "Icy Tubes" range is really refreshing in the hot weather as you can put the products in the fridge and their "Ultra Shiny Sun Lip Gloss" is great for the delicate skin of the mouth.

NIVEA and JOHNSON'S are cheaper alternatives and their high SPF sunscreen products are good for all ages and skin types. The most sensually pleasurable sun protection product I have found is JOHNSON'S SUN CARE KIDS Hydrating Sun Protection Lotion (SPF 35) which smells divinely of apricots, to such an extent that even children actually enjoy putting it on. If only good old HAWAIIAN TROPIC would manufacture products with a higher SPF factor: the HT scent is a true sense sensation, smelling as it does of Piña Coladas. I suppose we will just have to stick with real Piña Coladas on the beach but in moderation, please, ladies!

If you are a brunette or a redhead you will probably look great with pale, creamy skin but most blondes seem to prefer the sun-kissed look. Whatever your hair colour a deep, golden tan will cover a multitude of sins including fat, cellulite, stretch marks et al; everyone seems to look slimmer and healthier with a tan. In the twenty-first century it is no problem achieving the golden goddess look without going near the sun. Fake tans are now simply brilliant and orange palms, streaks and splodges should be a thing of the past.

Tanning

However if you are nervous about applying a fake tan yourself go to a salon and get yourself professionally sprayed; spray tans are really cheap and cheerful nowadays. The best one in Central London is THE TANNING SHOP in Kensington (4 Campden Hill Road, Kensington High Street, W8 7DU, phone 020 7938 1932) run by mother and daughters team Margaret, Annie and Lara. Their spray tan is called "Mystic Tan": you stand in a booth and are sprayed from top to toe, front and back in just one minute. There are three levels of colour to suit all skin types and the tan is completely natural looking. THE TANNING SHOP'S satisfied customers include ROBBIE WILLIAMS and GERI HALLIWELL: we did actually run into ROBBIE emerging from the shop once and chased him down the road until he agreed to give my daughter JADE his autograph on my cheque book! But I digress…. Annie at THE TANNING SHOP says *"do not shower for twenty four hours after your Mystic Tan and do not go to the gym immediately afterwards or you will sweat it off! The fake tan usually lasts at least five days depending on how often you bath, shower, swim, etc.*

Perhaps you would prefer to be tanned "in the comfort of your own home"? There are various professional spray tanners who will in fact come to you with their little machines, including fast and accurate sprayer LAURA FERRALL-PEEVEY (07867 610 045, www.bronzetallulah.co.uk). Laura's system is called an "Air Brush Tan" and uses an American product called "Totally Tan" in a spray gun which gives the skin a lovely golden colour. It takes twenty minutes to apply to your whole body and fifteen minutes for a half body, then a further ten minutes to dry. Laura says *"the advantage of my system is that you can personalise your tan by building it up in some areas more than others. For instance the chest area is usually the hardest to tan so you can have two or three layers there. You can also have less layers on your face for a more natural look. Do not shower for twelve hours after spraying and use plenty of moisturiser to keep the fake tan going. It should last for at least a week".*

Laura also has her own BRONZE TALLULAH spray tanning shop in Brixton at 88 Atlantic Road, SW9 8PX, phone 020 7733 5588.

Whatever sort of spray tan you have, booth or gun, there are two areas you will need to watch: your hands and your feet. Put plenty of barrier cream or moisturiser between your fingers and toes, round your nails and on the backs of your wrists and your heels. Wash these areas about one and a half to two hours after your spray, leaving the rest of you to "take" for a minimum of four hours or overnight if more convenient. Then your hands and feet will not be browner than everywhere else which is always a dead giveaway!

Once you have got the fake tan bug you will definitely want to maintain it: looking like a sun goddess all year round is now so easy. You will not believe that you used to cook yourself for hours in the sun getting hot and sticky and ruining your skin. But even if you are tanned professionally on a regular basis, there will be times when you will need to apply fake tan yourself if you want to keep up the bronzed look. For instance your fake tan will fade much more quickly in the pool or the sea on holiday, which is just where you need it most. So always take a big supply of fake tan with you for topping up every day or so.

Get into the habit of exfoliating thoroughly before each professional fake tan or once a week if you are a do it yourself tanner. If you use ST TROPEZ, the famous original fake tan, you will be able to buy their own brand exfoliant and after tan moisturiser. Or use a good exfoliant like THE SANCTUARY's "Body Scrub" and apply it with exfoliating gloves (available from SALLY'S Beauty Supply shops nationwide). Once your skin is fresh and pale again you are ready for your fake tanning session, whether at home or at a salon. You should exfoliate all over once a week anyway even if you are not using fake tans; your skin will feel much softer and smoother. After your tanning session moisturise thoroughly every morning and night to keep your newly bronzed skin glowing.

Fake tanning products

The amount of fake tans on the market is quite frightening but some are much better than others. If you have a steady hand go for a spray tan which is the fastest method of tanning; the best ones I have reviewed for HOT GOSSIP are LANCÔME's "Flash Bronzer Self Tanning Dry Body Oil" which is self explanatory and gives a lovely shimmery look, BOOTS' "Soltan Self Tan Spray" which is very fast drying and cheap and SKIN DOCTORS' "Jungle Bronze Self Tanning Spray", available from BOOTS and large department stores, which is also reasonable and gives a very deep tan.

If you prefer to use a mousse which you can rub in, try the ST TROPEZ Mousse or MAXITAN "Self Tanning Lotion", a fantastic vanilla flavoured mousse product available exclusively from 020 7938 1152.

Gel products are slightly harder to apply but work really well on small areas like the face, neck and décolleté. LANCÔME's "Flash Bronzer Self-Tanning Face Gel" gives a beautiful natural colour to these areas and lasts very well.

The only self tanning milk I have found is CLARINS' "Liquid Bronze Self Tanning" for the face, neck and décolleté which glides on easily, smells very fresh and gives a deep tan with just one application. As this product is a milk, do not forget to shake it well before applying as the colouring agent can separate.

Nothing looks worse than the "you've been tangoed" orange look so go easy on the fake tanning when you start. If you are at all doubtful about the outcome on your particular skin tone, always apply moisturiser first for a paler, more natural looking "sun kiss".

Every now and then all we fake tanners will get caught out in our natural white and pasty state. But there is never any need to turn down a hot date just because you are less than tanned at the time. SKIN DOCTORS' JUNGLE BRONZE "Bronzing Skin Gloss" is a temporary tanning cream which you can rub in to your whole body in five minutes to give a you a gorgeous coffee colour with sparkles which will not come off when swimming or playing sport but does wash off easily with soap. This creamy gloss glides on easily and you can build it up with two or three coats if you wish. Plus its tropical coconut smell is absolutely divine: like Hawaiian Tropic, I sometimes carry a tin of the Jungle Bronze Gloss around with me just to inhale it when I need a natural safe mood elevator! The JUNGLE BRONZE Gloss is one of my all time favourite HOT GOSSIP Products of the Month (phone 0800 298 9600 for stockists).

Sight

14

BEAUTY
THE SERIOUS STUFF

I F you have abused your skin for years in the sun or you are of a certain age or your skin care regime does not seem to be enough any more, you will probably think about Botox and "fillers". Everyone seems to be "at it" these days with Botox, even young people in their twenties. We all know that prevention is better than cure but the earlier you start these procedures the more time you will be spending getting yourself maintained rather than getting on with your life. Never forget that Botox is a type of poison and can have an adverse effect if injected in the wrong place. Plus you can have allergic reactions to some of the "fillers" such as Collagen, Hydrafill, Restylane, Perlane, etc. It is absolutely imperative that you go to a proper clinic and are treated by trained medical therapists, especially in the case of Botox where only a doctor or nurse should inject you. So forget the Botox parties and quick "lip jobs" in your lunch hour and do *not* drink alcohol before, during or after these sorts of serious injectable treatments.

Botox
Here is a quick run down of all the latest beauty procedures from beauty expert SIDRA SHAUKAT who is herself an advocate of natural beauty but admits that many ladies just want a "quick fix":

BOTOX AND OTHER BEAUTY PROCEDURES
from Sidra Shaukat

Botox
Botox injections have become the buzzword in beauty circles for women (and men!) who want to look as young as possible and not have frown lines on the forehead and nose to mouth lines. When patients who received Botox injections for facial tics noticed that it smoothed their facial lines, doctors realised they were onto a gold mine. Botox is now regularly used to eliminate certain wrinkles, such as the furrows from muscles in the forehead or near the eyes.

By using Botox to relax these muscles temporarily, or paralyse them if you want to use a scarier word, you make the wrinkles go away. Is it dangerous? Doctors say the diluted solution is safe if used properly. It can cost hundreds to thousands of pounds a year to keep up the look. Botox is proving so popular that the manufacturer sold enough for half a million doses.

Skin lasers
If you want a more lasting effect over the entire face, the latest treatment is laser. The idea with this is to moderately burn the skin so that it heals like new. The treatment, costing thousands, is so severe that even experts urge caution.

Chemical peels
Dermatologists use acids such as lactic, glycolic and salicylic acids, to chemically peel the skin and remove wrinkles and scars.

Collagen
Collagen, usually sterilised bovine collagen, is injected just beneath the skin to reduce the appearance of wrinkles. It is temporary and must be repeated every several months.

Dermabrasion
Dermabrasion is a surgical process where the skin is resurfaced by a rapidly rotating abrasive tool, such as a wire brush or ser-

rated wheel to produce a smoother complexion. Also used to get rid of acne scars.

Lunchtime peels

Many dermatologists offer peels that are so quick and mild that they can be done in a lunch hour. One popular type is particle resurfacing where a vacuum moves microscopic crystals over the skin, removing the outer layer. Lunchtime peels will not affect wrinkles, but are intended to fade sunspots and improve the skin.

Soft-tissue facial implants

Soft pliable synthetic material is surgically implanted under the skin to smooth wrinkles or furrows by providing support under the skin. They are most effective around the lips and mouth and can be used to fill in depressed scars.

Alpha and beta hydroxy acids

Hydroxy acids are used to peel off the top layers of the skin, improving its texture and colour. Alpha and beta hydroxy acids are in numerous cosmetics.

EVOLENCE

Let us go into more detail about "injectables". London's "Botox queen" SISTER MALTI O'MAHONY of THE BOSTON AESTHETICS CLINIC is one of the leading injectables practitioners in the UK and is often asked to correct bad Botox jobs. SISTER O'MAHONY is now using the latest and longest lasting injectable, EVOLENCE, and says of this new "wonder product":

EVOLENCE is a new, collagen-based; soft-tissue filler that quickly and effectively restores shape to facial wrinkles – with benefits lasting for at least 12 months.

EVOLENCE is a breakthrough in the treatment of the effects of ageing and in correcting lines and wrinkles. For the first time you can choose a totally natural solution that does not need costly repeat treatment every few months. EVOLENCE is for people who care about how they want to bring back the structure of much younger skin.

EVOLENCE is derived from the most "biocompatible" sources. This means that we select collagen that most closely resembles human tissue and is therefore very unlikely to cause any adverse reaction or be "rejected" by the body. We use the same biological source material that has been used in heart, dental and eye surgery for decades. EVOLENCE is made from porcine.

No one else has managed to "harness nature" in quite this way with Glymatrix technology. First we break down the source material into pure collagen molecules. Then we re-create the strong, long-lasting bonds that exist in nature using a naturally occurring sugar, ribose. The result is a collagen substantial enough to fill even deep facial contours instantly but with a low viscosity making it easy to inject.

EVOLENCE has an excellent safety profile. The injections produce some mild discomfort that is easily controlled with a local anaesthetic. A few patients may experience mild swelling or itching for a few days after injection.

EVOLENCE is intended for the correction of: Wrinkles; nasolabial folds; scars; atrophy from disease or trauma; defects secondary to rhinoplasty, skin graft or other surgically-induced irregularities; other soft tissue defects or deficiencies.

What distinguishes EVOLENCE from other injectable products?

While biodegradable dermal fillers are characterised by a limited short-term durability requiring repeat injections 2–3 times a year and synthetic products have disadvantages (e.g. unfavourable safety) associated with the permanency of their effects, EVOLENCE has taken the established safety profile of collagen and – by overcoming the limitation of its rapid biodegradability through Glymatrix technology (a novel cross-linking procedure) – has set a new standard in biodegradable facial filler technology with an effect lasting at least 12 months.

Is the pre-test necessary?

EVOLENCE is a natural product and due to the Glymatrix technology it is able to mimic the properties of the natural collagen found in the skin. Therefore, while an allergic reaction is theoretically possible, it is extremely rare. Pre-testing is not a prerequisite to treatment. Patients with a history of hypersensitivity and particularly known allergies to collagen should consult their doctor.

What is the origin?

The highly purified collagen used in the manufacture of EVOLENCE is derived from porcine tendons. Due to their high degree of immunocompatibility, porcine collagen materials are favoured for use in human medicine, e.g. heart valve replacement, corneal shields, implantable lenses, wound dressing in burn therapy, surgical membranes and surgical mesh patches for tissue repair.

Precautions

Should only be injected into skin which is free from inflammation and infection.

As with any injection, patients using substances which may reduce coagulation, such as aspirin and non-steroidal anti-inflammatory drugs, may experience increased bruising or bleeding at the injection site.

Not recommended for use in periorbital area.

Other collagen fillers have shown that over correction of the vermillion border of the lip has been slow to resolve due to minimal tissue stresses at this site. Therefore, caution is advised when using EVOLENCE in this area.

EVOLENCE should be used with caution in patients on immunosuppressive therapy or those with known connective tissue diseases.

It is recommended that the use of EVOLENCE collagen implants in individual patients be limited to 10 ml over a one-year period.

Is EVOLENCE for anyone?

EVOLENCE is contraindicated in the following: Patients with

- known hypersensitivity to any collagen products
- a history of anaphylactic reactions or serious recurrent allergic reactions
- undergoing or planning to undergo desensitisation injections to porcine meat products, as these injections can contain porcine collagen
- pregnant and lactating women.

Aquamid

SISTER O'MAHONY told me that the one area which is really difficult to "fill" because it really does not last is the mouth. She said: *"I am now using Aquamid, a safe water-based gel, on the lips because it usually lasts for four to five years".*

"Aquamid™ is injected under the skin as a soft filling with a fine needle. Together with the practitioner you can decide, in front of the mirror, what the final cosmetic results should be: what you see is what you get. The procedure is quick, needs neither hospitalisation nor general anaesthetic and does not need recovery time and gives hardly any discomfort. After the injection you can go home or back to work immediately.

Aquamid™ is a revolutionary novelty on the world market, has previously been thoroughly tested over ten years on more than 30,000 patients. It has proved to be an effective and absolutely safe product. Clinical trials in Europe have proved that any side effects are few and harmless. At first, the corrected area may be a little swollen, but this usually subsides spontaneously after 1–2 days.

Aquamid™ is developed and manufactured in Denmark to the highest international standards of quality and safety control (www.aquamid.nl)."

ALL ABOUT BOTOX

Regarding Botox, SISTER O'MAHONY told me everything you could ever wish to know about this extraordinary treatment and here it is:

As a convenient alternative to surgery, for younger patients it is possible to use injections of a substance called Botox to reduce and relax frown lines, forehead lines and even laughter lines around the eyes. The benefits of Botox injections are visible within five days of the treatment and will last for 3–6 months, giving the face a smoother, more rested appearance. After this period, the benefits of Botox will still be visible as wrinkles and lines will be diminished. If a more permanent look is required, the furrows may be filled with Hydra Fill, Aquamid, Evolence, Restylane or Sculptra.

How do the Botox injections work?

They are produced from botulinum toxin, which temporarily relaxes the muscles into which it is injected. Because facial expressions result in wrinkling or furrowing – especially on the forehead and around the eyes – Botox prevents you from making these expressions so that the skin around the injection site stays smooth.

How was it discovered that Botox could achieve these smoothing effects?

Botox has been used successfully for a number of years to treat people with serious nervous ticks and facial spasms. The smoothing effect of the Botox injections was noticed around the injection sites and as a result, cosmetic surgeons perfected the treatment of lines around the forehead and eyes.

Which are the best areas of the face for Botox treatment?

The vertical frown lines between the eyes, around the laughter lines and the horizontal lines on the forehead.

Are Botox injections painful?

The pain factor is minimal – you will feel a pinprick at the injection followed by a mild burning sensation that wears off in minutes.

Will there be a long term benefit to having Botox injections?

Yes, by preventing the muscles from moving for a period of time, your lines will be diminished and will appear less marked.

What should I do after my Botox injections have worn off?

A return treatment will maintain your smooth new look.

Is Botox safe?

The botolinum toxin in the Botox injections is sterile, safe and has been used for over ten years to treat serious medical conditions.

How long will the Botox treatment take?

Your clinic will advise you as to how many injections you will require and where they will be placed. Usually Botox treatments take about 15 minutes to perform.

How will I look after the Botox injections?

You may have a few tiny pink marks where the injections were made but these will disappear within two days. Most people are able to immediately return to a normal life after the treatment.

Can I have my Botox injections done in my lunchtime?

Yes, this is one of the new non-surgical procedures, which is ideally suited to "lunch-time treatments". You will certainly be able to return to work.

Are there any activities I should avoid after my treatment?

Avoid lying down for a few hours and keep the head upright to keep the solution from travelling to other areas. Avoid activities such as shoe shopping and yoga. The full effects will take at least five days to develop.

Are there any side effects to this treatment?

If the injection sites are placed too close to the eye then an eyebrow droop can occur. Likewise, if too much Botox is injected into one spot this can hinder facial expressions.

Patients with thicker more elastic skin will respond well to being relaxed.

Who are the best candidates for this treatment?

Anyone, female or male who wishes to look more rested. Ideal candidates are younger patients with thicker more elastic skin who will respond well to being relaxed.

Botox really is remarkable stuff and can even be injected in the armpits and in the palms of the hands to stop you perspiring in those areas, which is great news if you have this unfortunate problem. Some ladies have even tried having their décolletés Botoxed although I cannot personally see how this works as I have never noticed any muscles to "paralyse" in the area between the boobs! "Fillers?" Yes, that makes total sense if you have fine lines or wrinkles in that area.

Cutera lasers

THE BOSTON AESTHETICS CLINIC treats half the celebs in London and MALTI told me that the clinic's other most popular treatments at the moment are acupuncture, sclerotherapy (the treatment of thread veins with the powerful CUTERA "Coolglide" laser), laser hair removal (with the same machine), "Mesolift" (injections of a cocktail of vitamins, minerals and amino acids into the facial skin to give a more youthful and radiant appearance) and microdermabrasion (which involves spraying the skin with fine crystals to "resurface" or peel the top layer and reveal the fresh young skin underneath). Microdermabrasion is currently the Big One for freshening up the face, décolleté and hands.

Cynosure lasers

The face, décolleté and hands are areas where "age spots" or "pigmentation" can show up once you reach the grand old age of thirty or so. "Photo Rejuvenation" is a (newish) laser treatment specifically for "photo damaged" skin, i.e. skin which has been over exposed to the sun's ultra violet rays, causing coarsening of the skin texture, wrinkling and irregular pigmentation. Most ladies of over 30 who lead an active lifestyle will be affected and sadly it does not improve with age! The CYNOSURE lasers used by many of the top clinics for Photo Rejuvenation are fast, powerful and gentle and the "zapping with white light" treatment, as some clients call it, is not too painful. Usually a few treatments will completely get rid of nasty brown "pigmentation" marks to give a much more even and youthful appearance to the skin.

Medical therapist JOANNE EVANS, the skin care specialist at The Medical Rooms at The Soma Centre (2–24 High Street Kensington, W8 4TP, phone 020 7361 0616/07710 381 438) is one of London's most enthusiastic Photo Rejuvenation practitioners and reports great success with the procedure at her clinic.

Anti-ageing

JOANNE undertakes all the usual facial, hair removal, etc. treatments at The Soma Centre as well as some really interesting anti-ageing specialities including:

- ❧ "Dr Schrammek GreenPeel": a herbal peel using plant extracts
- ❧ "Environ Vitamin facials"
- ❧ "Mini lift": a quick fix for a special occasion
- ❧ "Aurora Glow": a really adventurous facial featuring an enzymatic peel, impulse light and Royal Honey (very DAME BARBARA CARTLAND!)

INTENSE PULSED LIGHT TREATMENT

One treatment which is really good for sun damaged skin and age spots as well as the dreaded red veins on the face is Intense Pulsed Light Treatment (IPL). This practically painless laser treatment usually requires around 2–4 sessions and you can have it with CLARE ROBSON, my favourite therapist at the respected DR PATRICK BOWLER's COURT HOUSE CLINIC in Wimpole Street. Here is some bumph on IPL:

What is an Intense Pulsed Light (IPL) Treatment?

IPL Treatment is a series of gentle pulsed light treatments intended to improve the appearance of sun damaged and aged skin, as well as reduce redness and flushing. IPL treatments result in a more youthful-appearing skin. They have been developed to consistently and predictably improve the visible appearance of the skin without needing lots of time away from work.

What are the causes of red faces?

Literally millions of people in the UK have an undesirable redness and/or sun damage of the face. The more common causes are Rosacea (a condition in up to 13 million people), sun exposure, alcohol, medications, stress, emotional causes, time and ageing of the skin and repeated blushing or flushing of the skin as seen most commonly in fair skinned individuals of northern European descent.

How does the treatment work?

An intense light is emitted in a series of gentle pulses over the skin at regular intervals for a treatment course as decided by your doctor. This special light which is different from laser treatments emits light over many wavelengths allowing the light to penetrate to all the levels of the skin where abnormal and easily dilated vessels can be found. (Lasers produce only a single wavelength of light and are limited in depth of penetration and in what they can treat). On average 90% improvement is seen in most patients.

Are there any other conditions that can be treated with the IPL?

Yes. IPL treatments will also help patients who suffer from photo-ageing of the skin, pigmentation from sun exposure (Age Spots) and irregularities of skin texture.

Titan procedure

At the time of writing CUTERA, the big American laser company were conducting trials on "Titan", a new procedure which they described as "the first light-based solution for tightening skin". ("Titan"/tighten: geddit?) CUTERA reported great success with the procedure in the US and their "before and after" stomach close ups of a 50 year old patient with "postpartum skin redundancy" (basically getting saggy baggy after pregnancy and childbirth) were extraordinary.

The Titan Procedure uses an infrared light source to tighten the skin and stimulate collagen re-growth and can be used on the face and neck as well as all over the body. It is an uncomfortable treatment like most of the ones that really work (Botox, "fillers", Mesotherapy, etc.) but apparently gets amazing results after just one session, although a course is recommended. If the trials prove successful, the Titan Procedure will be available from MR MICHAEL BOWEN, FRCS, MCOG (Ire) (10 Harley Street, London, W1G 9PF, phone 020 7467 8471).

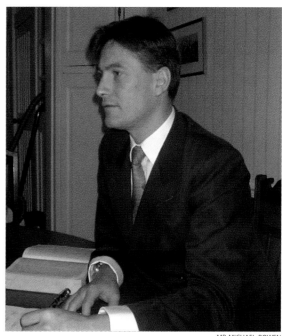

MR MICHAEL BOWEN

Sight

15

ALTERNATIVE
HEALTH TREATMENTS

THE BOSTON CLINIC's sister establishment, THE BOSTON OPTIMUM HEALTH CLINIC (George St, London, W2, phone 020 7935 7789) and THE HALE CLINIC (7 Park Crescent, London W1, phone 020 7631 0156) offer colonic irrigation (colon hydrotherapy) a much-maligned deep cleansing and purifying treatment for the intestines, beloved of PRINCESS DIANA. People usually say "yuk" when they hear the words "colonic irrigation" but the treatment is painless and actually quite relaxing as well as extremely effective. If you have digestive problems, want to be your thinnest possible or just want to feel healthy and re-energised internally, give it a shot. As SOPHIE ANDERTON memorably remarked in "I'M A CELEBRITY – GET ME OUT OF HERE", "you can have twenty year old faeces in your gut" and who in their right mind really needs that? Below is a report from THE HALE CLINIC on "colonics".

THE HALE CLINIC is one of London's leading "alternative therapy" clinics and gave me the following comprehensive list of some of the interesting treatments you can now have at their and other alternative clinics (besides colonic irrigation and kinesiology which we mentioned previously) and what exactly they comprise:

COLONIC IRRIGATION
from The Hale Clinic

Colon hydrotherapy or irrigation is a gentle infusion of warm, purified water that can help eliminate mucus, stored waste matter and toxins from the bowel. The colon forms the last part of the digestive tract. Its function is to absorb the water-soluble nutrients as well as synthesise certain vitamins. It is also a major player in the excretory system responsible for eliminating food and other wastes when the internal environment becomes unbalanced due to stress, food additives, certain drugs, smoking and excess alcohol.

Who can benefit from this therapy?
- Anyone suffering from irritable bowel system (IBS)
- Patients with chronic constipation
- Those wishing to embark on a detoxification program
- Patients with Candida and yeast infections

What is involved?
A detailed case history is taken followed by an explanation of the procedure. The Colonic itself takes between 30–45 minutes during which time water will be gently introduced into the colon via the rectum whilst the therapist uses special massage techniques to stimulate the release of stored matter. Your modesty is preserved at all times.

This treatment can also indicate the presence of parasites and whether the patient has difficulty in breaking down certain proteins and carbohydrates or whether too much mucus is being produced.

- ACUPRESSURE *A natural healing technique that uses applied pressure to relevant points on the body releasing blockages*
- ACUPUNCTURE
- ALEXANDER TECHNIQUE
- ALLERGY CLINIC *Testing for inhalant allergies and food intolerances*
- ANTHROPOSOPHIC MEDICINE *complementary approach using also homeopathic and herbal remedies for mind, body and spirit treatment*
- AROMATHERAPY *Fragrant oils that have healing properties are massaged into the skin*
- AURA-SOMA COLOUR *Gifts, talents and challenges revealed through rainbow coloured healing oils*
- AUTISM INTEGRATED APPROACH *Using brain wave/music, homoeopathic removal of the side effects of vaccinations, desensitisation to dramatically enhance the body's own healing ability*
- AYURVEDA *Ancient Indian form of medicine/treatment relying on herbal remedies, massage, yoga and meditation*
- BICOM RESONANCE *An innovative holistic medicine technique. The Bicom device both diagnoses and treats the health problem*
- BIO-ENERGY HEALING *The healer acts as a channel allowing positive energy to pass through the patient with one hand and extracting negative energy with the other*
- C.A.C.I. *Non-surgical face lift that restores strength to muscles through electronic stimulation*
- CANCER SUPPORT CLINIC
- CHAKRA BALANCING *A traditional holistic healing process for the relief of back, joint and other physical, emotional and spiritual pains*
- CHINESE HERBAL MEDICINE *Complete health system that looks at the body as a balance between the opposite energies of yin and yang*
- CHIROPODY/PODIATRY *Food care treatment for sports injuries, foot and back pain, etc.*
- CHIROPRACTIC *Manual treatment of musculo-skeletal aches and pains*
- COSMETIC ACUPUNCTURE *The Japanese tradition offers a unique holistic anti-ageing treatment that encourages the natural ability of the skin to heal itself*
- DEEP TISSUE MASSAGE *A preventative treatment that works on neuro-muscular tissues strengthening the nervous system*
- EAR CONING *Relieves pressure, fights infection and gently removes toxins and excess wax from the ears improving hearing, vision, taste, smell and balance*

- "EMDR" *Eye movement technique that stimulates the mind to remove stress and traumas*
- ENERGY HEALING *A form of energy transference that corrects the body's aura – effective for chronic fatigue syndrome, stroke and cancer patients*
- GENERAL MEDICAL SCREENING
- HERBAL MEDICINE
- HOMOEOPATHY *Remedies derived from mineral, plant and animal sources that stimulate the body's own healing mechanism*
- JIN SHIN JYUTSU *Powerful Japanese method of repairing physical, mental and emotional stress*
- JUNGIAN PSYCHOTHERAPY *Addresses client's stress, depression, addiction/alcohol, relationship and work problems, infertility and bereavement in a solution-oriented way*
- LIA THERAPY *Transforms the skin making the face look immediately younger and skin tighter and rejuvenated*
- LOMI LOMI MASSAGE *A magical healing massage derived from Ancient Polynesia that promotes balance and harmony allowing change by connecting Mind, Body and Spirit*
- MIND PURIFICATION *Secret ritual of massage therapy in ancient medicine – over 5,000 years old – gives peace and purifies the mind*
- NATURAL BREAST ENHANCEMENT *Through hypnosis*
- NATUROPATHY *Treats the underlying cause of illness not just the symptoms*
- NET THERAPY *Normalises unresolved physical and/or behaviour patterns of the body*
- NLP *Neurolinguistic programming is a powerful form of brief psychotherapy that taps into the subconscious breaking destructive behaviour patterns and enabling transformation to take place*
- NUTRITION
- ORTHOPAEDIC MEDICINE
- OSTEOPATHY
- PERIODONTAL DISEASE THERAPY *Heals damage done to gum tissue and bone by infection and protects general health from invasive micro-organisms*
- POLARITY THERAPY *A powerful holistic energy medicine that uses a combination of bodywork, stretching exercises, cleaning diets and health awareness to assist the body's own healing process*
- REFLEXOLOGY *Massage the pressure points in the hands and feet which correspond to different parts of the body providing overall relaxation*
- REIKI *It can help restore and balance energy, reducing stress and aiding spiritual growth*

☙ REJUVANESSENCE *Dubbed the "fingertip face lift", the therapist gently manipulates the facial and scalp muscles helping to re-tone and re-shape form and improve circulation*

☙ ROLFING *Method of manipulating the body's muscles, fascia and connective tissue to align the whole structure and free it from chronic tension*

☙ SERVICE FOR CHILDREN *Offers complementary treatment for children and adolescents and advice for parents and carers provided by an experienced medical doctor and, where appropriate, an interdisciplinary team of therapists*

☙ SHEN THERAPY *Helps whenever your emotions hold you back in life. Clients report rapid recovery from childhood emotional, physical and sexual abuse or other traumas*

☙ SHYNESS COUNSELLING

☙ SPORTS PHYSICIAN

☙ STRESS MANAGEMENT

☙ TRAGER *Mind and body re-education therapy suitable for a wide range of conditions from carpal tunnel syndrome to Parkinson's disease*

☙ TRICHOLOGY

☙ TUNA MASSAGE *A Chinese therapeutic massage to regulate the function of internal organs which helps with the recovery of injured muscles, tendons, bones and joints*

☙ WEIGHT REDUCTION

THE HALE CLINIC also offers a telephone advisory service so that you can decide exactly which treatments will benefit you most.

As you can see, the amount of "alternative" health treatments now available is mind-boggling. Apart from the famous clinics such as the ones I have mentioned, how do you know who is good and who is not? I normally feel safe if I hear that a clinic is By Royal Appointment. THE GEMELLE CLINIC at London's DORCHESTER HOTEL is not exactly By Royal Appointment but it does have Royal patronage, inasmuch as I was told PRINCE PHILIP is a client along with sports stars such as ANNA KOURNIKOVA and AUDREY HARRISON and film stars PIERCE BROSNAN and BILLY ZANE.

Run by twins STEFANIA and DONATA D'ADDETTA, GEMELLE's star therapist is ALESSANDRA CAPPONI (07930 481 869) who practices shiatsu, reflexology, aromatherapy and Ayurvedic massage, as well as cranial sacral therapy and crystal therapy. I actually tried the last three therapies with ALESSANDRA myself and found them most beneficial.

If you live in Essex, one natural health practitioner who is also a healer and is highly regarded is LORAINE MEYERS (Harmony House, Colchester Road, Chappel, Colchester, CO6 2AB, phone 01206 247 178, lmeyers3490@aol.com). LORAINE is a life coach, reflexologist, kinesiologist, nutritionist and neuro-linguistic practitioner (NLP). She also teaches and gives Reiki, treats skin conditions and offers an Ayurvedic "face lift" which is very popular.

Sight

16

BEAUTY
EVEN MORE SERIOUS STUFF

Back on the serious beauty beat DR LUCY GLANCEY tells us about her two latest and greatest facial procedures, ISOLAGEN and THREAD LIFTING (more details overleaf).

"We are living in times when our attitude to how we look is changing rapidly. Up till not long ago any treatment aimed at improving one's looks was considered mere vanity. Now it is not unusual to combine one's weekly facial with four-monthly Botox or six monthly dermal filler injections.

The so called lunchtime procedures have revolutionalised our current concept of a beauty treatment and have bridged the gap between beauty therapy and cosmetic surgery. These comprise a large group of treatments: Botulinum toxin injections, dermal fillers, subdermal fillers, chemical peels, lasers, sclerotherapy, mesotherapy, thread lift, Isolagen and new ones are coming on the market rapidly."

If you are that bit older and/or feel that Botox and fillers are not enough for you or if you have certain features that you want to change, you may wish to consider cosmetic surgery. Surgery is a big deal, involving anaesthesia and, usually, actual cutting. There is always a risk with any kind of surgery or anaesthetic and the cost of "plastic aesthetic" surgery is often prohibitive so think carefully before embarking on this course. We are lucky that we now live in an age where if you do not like your features you can change them and if you do not like growing older you can arrest the wrinkles.

The cosmetic surgeons are truly playing God and can usually change people's lives for the better. But some patients become hooked on the surgery and go over the top; for instance MICHAEL JACKSON looked perfect in his "THRILLER" era in 1984 but now sadly he looks very strange

after allegedly having further operations. You absolutely do not want to achieve a "BRIDE OF WILDENSTEIN" look and it is imperative that you go to a reputable cosmetic surgeon. This kind of surgery is quite acceptable in today's world and there is no need to feel embarrassed.

You will need to be referred by your GP so consult him or her first and, if necessary, go to see various surgeons before deciding which one is for you. Alternatively contact cosmetic surgery guru CINDY JACKSON (www.cindyjackson.com) who will advise you on both cosmetic surgeons and surgery. You can also purchase CINDY's fascinating books, *Cosmetic Surgery Secrets* (which is updated every three months) and her autobiography *Living Doll* from her website. CINDY has herself had over forty cosmetic surgery procedures since 1988 and now looks absolutely superb, often being mistaken for German supermodel CLAUDIA SCHIFFER. However CINDY had this succinct comment for readers: "be b... careful! And, however careful you are, cosmetic surgery can still go wrong". So, ladies, straight from the horse's mouth: in other words approach this type of surgery with the utmost caution. You must find the best possible surgeon and expect to pay big bucks: cosmetic surgery is absolutely not something you can skimp on.

When we think about cosmetic surgery for maintenance, we think about the face lift but how does it actually work? Over to MR EDWARD LATIMER-SAYER who operates at HIGHGATE PRIVATE HOSPITAL (020 8341 4182) and THE BELVEDERE PRIVATE HOSPITAL (020 8311 4464). MR LATIMER-SAYER is known for his "heroic face lifts" and has had great success with older patients.

A SHORT HISTORY OF FACE LIFTING

from Mr Edward Latimer-Sayer

The first face lifts were done in the early years of the 20th century, round about 1903. The operation consisted of making a curved incision above the ear in the scalp and pulling the front edge of the incision upwards and backwards so it overlapped. The overlap was then cut off and the wound sewn up. This lifted the facial skin a bit – about the same amount as pulling the hair back in a ponytail!

Unfortunately the skin tends to stretch a bit and the scar widens over time and the results (never very dramatic) tend not to last. The development of the face lift incision for the next 40 years involved more and more radical undermining of the skin. While giving an effective face lift, if the skin was pulled a bit tight and if the operation was repeated too often, this could give rise to the "wind tunnel" over-operated look.

After the Second World War it was realised that it wasn't only the skin that was becoming lax but the muscles too tended to droop with age. In the 1950s the surgeons learned ways of pulling both the muscle and the skin. This was pioneered by Skoog in Scandinavia. The muscles involved are called the SMAS (subcutaneous muscu-loaponeurotic system). There are now many variants of SMAS lifts.

In the 1980s surgeons through their experience with liposuction realised that the fat was also drooping. They began removing the drooping fat from the jowl region before lifting the muscle and skin – then replacing it into those regions where the fat has been lost: the upper lip and the nasolabial folds.

Trying to implant fat has a long history. It fails when used to bulk out large areas (breast augmentation, buttock increase) because the implanted fat cannot find a blood supply and dies. However the blood supply is very rich in the face and the small amounts of fat required to make a differ-

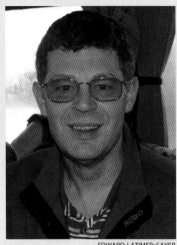

EDWARD LATIMER-SAYER

ence readily "take" as a graft and produce long-lasting results.

These days a modern surgeon will assess a patient's face and will decide what procedures need to be employed in any particular case. It is no longer true that one size fits all. Patients who have signifi-cant jowl formation will be treated with liposuction in the jowl region and the fat implanted into the upper lip and nasolabial creases and the muscles then lifted to their youthful position. The skin is then redraped gently over the rejuvenated face and does not need to be pulled too tight. Patients with very hollow cheeks are best treated by doubling over the SMAS to replace the lost bulk. Very wrinkled faces are still treated by the radical undermining of the skin proce-dure – the skin lift.

A face lift only lifts the mid and lower parts of the face and the neck. Over the last 20 years browlifts have become much more popular. The original method which involves a long incision over the top of the head still produces the most dramatic and long-lasting results. Many surgeons have opted for using an endoscope – small incisions in the scalp – and supporting the forehead skin on the skull bone.

Because a full face lift is pretty major surgery these days surgeons have gone back to just making a small incision around the ears and lifting the skin without much undermining. This can be done in a few minutes under local anaesthetic and is called a minilift – however, it does not last which is why this procedure was aban-doned in the first place. It is estimated that a minilift lasts as long as it takes the surgeon to spend the money…

Several attempts have been made to pro-duce the same effect as a face lift without major surgery by lifting the skin on hooks or suture material but they all suffer from rather temporary results. Similarly stimulat-ing the facial muscles to contract using an electrical device produces a short-term lift of the mid face but has no effect on skin laxity.

Overall the modern face lift is a very effective operation, so much so that the word has passed into general usage to mean any dramatic improvement in appearance and it is now applied (and overused) to a huge range of objects and even concepts.

THE ISOLAGEN AND THREAD LIFTING PROCEDURES

from Dr Lucy Glancey

Isolagen

One of the most exciting recent advances is Isolagen. It is not so much a procedure or a technique as a whole new concept – the so called self-rejuvenation. The process involves culturing the patient's own cells by removing a tiny piece of skin (biopsy) which then gets sent to a laboratory. Usually the skin is removed from behind the ear as this is considered to be the most sun-naïve area i.e. an area that does not routinely get exposed to the sun and therefore has best quality skin cells. While this may be the case for most women a lot of men frequently have this area exposed and therefore the skin has to be collected from other places. The cells are processed in the laboratory and then either stored for future use or given back to the patient in the form of a liquid suspension for injection.

It is an idea that appeals to everyone; those who would never consider having any foreign material injected into their faces but would have their own cells, those who are still young but would like to freeze their cells while they are still equally young for future use and for those who are looking for a long lasting solution for their facial, neck and décolleté lines. Unlike the conventional dermal fillers which look best immediately after the procedure and then slowly decline in effect over the next 6–12 months Isolagen starts working from 6–12 weeks after the procedure with gradual improvement with the results lasting seven years and possibly longer. It not only plumps up lines but also achieves a skin tightening effect because of the new col-

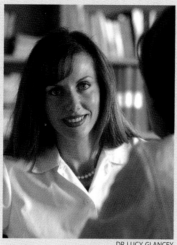

DR LUCY GLANCEY

lagen produced by the cultured skin cells. It is like planting seeds into the ground that later produce a bumper crop of the body's own collagen which is primarily important for maintaining the skin's elasticity.

Thread lift

Thread lift is one of the most logical procedures to have been developed – how many women say that they wished they could sellotape their excess facial skin behind their ears. The thread lift does exactly that. Surgical sutures are used to achieve lifting of various parts of the face and body. Because no skin is removed this technique is mostly suitable for the 35–50 age group. If you are older the excess skin will crease too much and become more noticeable. It can also be used in much younger individuals in which case it would not be a rejuvenation but a

beautification procedure i.e. it can achieve higher cheek bones or a more prominent chin in order to balance the profile.

High cheekbones have recently become very desirable. There are certain facial proportions which if present allow us to perceive a face as attractive. For example the two cheeks and chin should lie in the same plane which is known as the "beauty triangle" therefore increasing the volume of the cheek bones and chin has become a routine part of the so called tri-dimensional face lifting. The volume can be increased simply by injecting a volumising agent into the deep tissues (a specially formulated filler or the patient's own fat). Alternatively it can be achieved with the help of a thread lift procedure. There are two main types of threads in common use and each comes under many different commercial names. The first type is the barbed thread – it has tiny little barbs along its length which allows it to hold itself without any support just like a hold-up stocking. The other type of thread is smooth and therefore would require support (just like a stocking with a suspender). This support is usually a stable point in the tissues on which the thread is anchored.

Opposite he tells us everything we need to know about this extraordinary modern surgery which has ensured that our favourite film stars will always look gorgeous, young and reassuringly the same for their whole screen careers!

Two of TATLER's "World's Top Ten" cosmetic surgeons are in fact British and can be found in London's Harley Street: BARRY JONES and BASIM MATTI, MB ChB FRCS (30 Harley Street, London, W1G 9PW, phone 020 7637 9595, www.bmplasticsurgery.com) who is also HOT GOSSIP UK's consultant cosmetic surgeon. MR MATTI is known for his fantastically small and discreet scars, a big consideration if you are undertaking any kind of surgery. Overleaf is his report on cosmetic surgery or "aesthetic plastic surgery" as it is sometimes known (never forget the important reconstructive work that is achieved through plastic surgery, for instance for cancer and burns victims and for birth abnormalities).

COSMETIC SURGERY

from Mr Basim Matti

My main message to ladies considering cosmetic surgery is to choose your surgeon carefully. Secondly, whatever operation you choose to have, do not overdo it: a subtle enhancement is usually best and less noticeable. As with all operations there can be complications. Cosmetic surgery is no more painful than any other surgery: any post operative discomfort can easily be controlled by painkillers. The most uncomfortable operation is probably the tummy tuck and the least painful is rhinoplasty but most procedures do not hurt and the recovery period is relatively quick. Girls could consider having a rhinoplasty (nose job) from the age of 17 or 18 when their nose has finished growing and a breast augmentation (boob job) from 19 or 20 when the breasts have stopped growing, but only if they are emotionally mature enough to handle the surgery.

The oldest lady I have operated on was a face lift patient of 84: this is quite safe as long as the patient is fit and healthy. I do not usually recommend starting maintenance surgery until the late 30s or early 40s. Before that I use fillers, Restylane being my favourite as it has the least side effects. I approve of Botox which can be started at a younger age; It is particularly successful on the forehead but also for around the eyes and mouth and on the neck. You should always take a conservative approach with Botox and be very careful around the delicate eye and mouth areas.

Microdermabrasion, which my nurse MELANIE carries out for me at my practice, has proved very successful for the face, hands and décolleté. In fact I would say it is the most successful treatment for the décolleté.

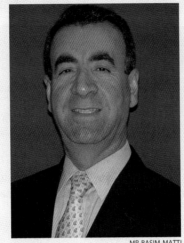

MR BASIM MATTI

When I perform a face lift it is very important to achieve harmony in the face. For this reason I like to do the whole face: brow, mid face and jowels, not forgetting the neck of course and I prefer to do the eyes at the same time. Otherwise the newly lifted areas can make the other areas look worse by comparison. The mid face is the most important area but the whole face must look harmonious.

You can do the eyes by themselves if you just have a bit of drooping above and/or puffiness below them. However you should not overdo the removal of fat from beneath the eyes as they will then tend to look sunken and haggard as you age.

You must not forget the rest of your body when you are having rejuvenating treatments, which is why I recommend microdermabrasion for the hands and décolleté. The hands are often a real giveaway and sometimes need more serious attention. My very latest operation is for the hands and involves autologous fat transfer (using your own fat, usually from the waist, tummy or knee) combined with vein removal. I weave the fat under the skin of the hands

and remove the more prominent veins, giving a much smoother, plumper and more youthful appearance to the hands. This operation is becoming increasingly popular: it is delicate to perform but can easily be done under local anaesthetic.

I suppose the most popular operations with me are face lifts, noses and breasts. Breast implants (prostheses) will always be popular; nowadays they can be inserted under the arm, through the nipple or under the bust and either behind or in front of the breast muscle. It is important to measure the width of the breast as well as the length before deciding on the size of prosthesis for the patient and she can choose either a round or a teardrop shaped implant. I also perform quite a lot of breast reductions and breast uplifts, both of which operations greatly improve a lady's natural bust line.

Liposuction and liposculpture are also popular at my practice. As sculpture is my hobby I find liposculpture very satisfying. The lateral waist, back, thighs, bottom, knees and abdomen all respond well to lipo.

For seriously large stomachs the abdominal lipectomy ("tummy tuck") is extremely effective but it leaves a large scar. I would say the least successful operations from my point of view as an aesthete are the arm and thigh lifts as there is no way of lifting these areas without making long incisions and therefore scars.

Scars, by the way, can be improved significantly by various methods. They can be injected with cortisone or you can use silicone gel or ointment or silicone "band aids" to thin them. I would have to inject the cortisone at my surgery but you can buy the silicone products at pharmacies over the counter.

ADVICE ON COSMETIC SURGERY

from Mr Alex Karidis

Perhaps you would like to look like your favourite celebrity. Well, wouldn't we all? However not even MR ALEX KARIDIS, MD FRCS (The Hospital of St John and St Elizabeth, 60 Grove End Road, London, NW8 9NK, phone 020 7432 8727, www.nip-ntuck.co.uk) who can spot a celeb's cosmetic surgery from photographs alone recommends this course. Popular TV and media cosmetic surgeon MR KARIDIS says "You have to think about your own natural height, shape and weight before slavishly copying someone else's looks. There is only so much a surgeon can do with the natural canvas". Here is MR KARIDIS' complete report:

I do not operate on many teenagers as they often are not psychologically mature enough to cope with the stress and discomfort of surgery. However the good news is that there is one cosmetic procedure which can be done at a very early age: girls can have their ears pinned back from as young as seven years old as the ears stop growing at this age.

At the other end of the scale I can go on performing face lifts on women up until the age of around 70 as long as the skin has not thinned too much by that age. Women can have more than one face lift in their lives: it depends on the individual. In fact I recommend that patients start earlier and maintain, little by little as they age, as I believe SOPHIA LOREN might have done as she still looks very good. *(Author's note: the pulchritudinous SOPHIA LOREN was voted "the most beautiful woman in the world" in 2004 at the age of 64, beating off all of her much younger rivals such as JULIA ROBERTS, CATHERINE ZETA-JONES. LIZ HURLEY, CLAUDIA SCHIFFER, et al.)*

If you leave it late like ANN ROBINSON or even JULIE CHRISTIE (who I think has now had

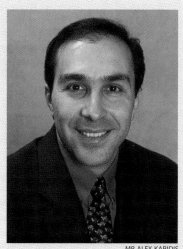

MR ALEX KARIDIS

two face lifts) it will be much more obvious and everyone will know you have had surgery. People still worry about being seen to have had cosmetic surgery: they do not want others to know and they do not want to appear vain. However I think this will change in the next 15 years or so and this sort of surgery will become far more accepted.

Before having a face lift you can try Botox and "fillers": there are now about 60 different types of fillers on the market. However I do not recommend the "permanent" fillers which last for up to five years as you cannot cut them out if you do not like them and the rest of your face changes naturally as you get older. For instance when LESLIE ASH had her famous "trout pout" lip job she would not have been able to have the filler removed without leaving scars on her lips. Under those circumstances you just have to wait for the filler to disappear of its own accord. At least if you have a bad Botox job it can be corrected.

Silicone cheek implants can move and may need to be removed. However liquid silicone, which some surgeons in other countries inject to plump up the face, is very difficult to remove if it moves. In fact liquid silicone has now been banned.

Breast implants are now made of silicone once again after a cancer scare was

disproved. However the prostheses are not liquid, they are a solid (though soft) "sac", will not leak and can be removed easily if necessary.

Breast augmentations are among my most popular operations. Apart from where the incisions should be placed (under arm, under bust or through the nipple) you have to decide where exactly to place the prostheses. If you have plenty of your own flesh you can have them in front of the muscle for a full, round effect. However if you are very thin and do not have much flesh to cover the edge of the prostheses you may get the "BECKHAM" or "coconut halves" effect which is very obvious.

Then you will need to have the implants placed behind the muscle for more coverage. This is more painful to recover from and looks obvious when you are working out your pecs, for instance but looks much more natural for the rest of the time. Alternatively you can go for a compromise and place the implants in the sub fascial layer, which is above the muscles but underneath another layer of breast tissue. Round implants will give you a fuller look for the tops of the breasts whereas the "teardrop" shape will give you more fullness in the lower breast for a more natural look. However the "teardrop" shape does not look so good if it moves around within the breast whereas the round shape looks the same whatever position it is in. Patients often ask to be made into a certain cup size but this is not practical. There are hundreds of different sizes of prostheses and I usually ask the patient to try them on inside their bras until they get the desired effect: slightly bigger, quite a lot bigger or hugely bigger! One point I would like to make is that most women do not wear the correct bra size anyway so how do they know what size they really want to be?

Another area which you can successfully build up with silicone implants is the nose, an operation which is popular with people of Asian, African and Caribbean descent. You can also build up the nose from the patient's own rib, ear or cartilage (autologous method). There is usually some degree of absorption and the implant may move so this operation sometimes has to be revised.

I personally do not perform "bum lifts" although I know they are very popular in South America, for instance. The methods are either to insert implants, which requires a certain amount of elasticity in the skin, or to cut and lift which leaves a big scar. Glamour model EMMA JONES says she has had her buttocks threaded and lifted with the thread but I cannot see how this could last long with the constant pressure of sitting on the bottom. If it sounds too good to be true – it usually is!

Liposuction and liposculpture are amongst my "top ops" (along with face lifts and breasts). Nowadays these procedures are

much improved and the canulars used to remove the fat are much finer. We now have Ultrasonic Liposuction which dissolves the fat before removing it and Power Assisted Liposuction where a motor vibrates the fat away rather than the surgeon having to really work at it manually. Lipo can damage the skin, however, so the surgeon has to be careful.

The operations I do not perform are the arm, thigh and full body lifts as they leave big scars. The full body lift is really drastic, where you lift the legs and buttocks right up into the waist like a pair of trousers! This is what SHARON OSBOURNE had. Under those circumstances, when someone has lost their full body weight, for instance, it is the only recourse as the skin would be so loose but the operation requires a whole team of surgeons and lasts several hours.

Of all the operations I perform I would say that noses, breasts and removing under eye bags are the most successful. It is always

good to keep the look as natural as possible so that others cannot spot what you have had done. The least successful procedures to my mind are removing lines and wrinkles from older faces, especially around the eyes. It just does not look natural if you try to erase all the laughter lines from that area – then how does anyone know when you are smiling? In general prevention is better than cure: lifestyle, nutrition and avoiding exposure to the sun are all important. Smoking is the worst thing you can do to your skin and dehydration is also bad, so drink plenty of water. Eat properly: dieting and attendant weight loss are bad for the elasticity of the skin, especially after a certain age. If you pay attention to all these things you will look younger for longer and will not have to come to see me so soon!

The bad news is that of all the cosmetic surgeons I interviewed (and only the very best got into the book!) not one of them had a surgical solution for cellulite. I suppose if you had the "full body lift" it would heave everything out of the way including cellulite and stretch marks but what drastic measures for a little bit of orange peel! It looks like the beauty therapists, aesthetic nurses and cosmetic doctors rather than the cosmetic surgeons have got this particular market cornered and we will all be maintaining our "dimple smoothing treatments" for ever (because cellulite has a nasty habit of returning).

If you want to know what you will look like before embarking on expensive cosmetic surgery you could try "photo imaging", a process which is exclusive in London to aesthetic plastic surgeon MR LUCIAN ION, FRCS (Plast) (129 Harley Street, London, W1, phone 020 7224 5434, www.aesthetic-plastic-surgery.co.uk). Below MR ION describes photo imaging:

"Photo imaging

One of the more recent developments in the field of cosmetic surgery is the use of computer simulation as an analysis and prediction tool. Dedicated software is available that enables clinicians to use digital or digitised photographs and manipulate shapes, contours and surface texture at the click of a button.

One of the primary targets of this approach is to allow patients to experiment on the photographs with regards to the desired change and to see whether their approach leads to a pleasing and balanced appearance. It also allows people that notice features they like on others, whether famous or not, to try and 'fit them on to their face' to see if the end-product looks like what they anticipated.

The other very relevant aspect is that computer simulation allows the practitioner to understand better what the patient would like to achieve and put together a treatment plan most likely to deliver 'the goods'. Without any doubt, this is not a very accurate process and the next step will probably be three-dimensional photography as well as the derived simulation. The most common areas of applicability for this technology are in rhinoplasty surgery, chin reshaping, fat transfer and liposuction. These operations generally contour transformations without involving skin texture changes for which the simulation is more basic.

How does photo imaging work? A photo is taken with a digital camera, fed into a computer and projected onto a large overhead plasma screen for both surgeon and patient to see. Then thanks to a sophisticated software programme, the relevant features are redrawn by the surgeon – in full consultation with the patient – and the necessary procedures to achieve the desired look discussed. Though the exact look projected onto the screen might not be achieved one hundred percent, it gives a reassuring guideline to anybody worried about how they'll look after the operation."

Sight

17

SIGHT
LOOKING AFTER YOUR EYES &
KEEPING THEM HEALTHY

BEAUTY may be in the eye of the beholder but how beautiful are your own eyes and how healthy are they? All the cosmetics in the world will not make your eyes look bright and sparkling if they are tired or, God forbid, infected. Your eyes may be the mirror of your soul but are they mirroring vibrant good health and that inner glow which makes them sparkle?

Eye care
If like me, you are susceptible to eye allergies, you must be super careful, especially in summer with all the pollen and dust in the air. Protect your eyes by wearing UVA and UVB resistant wraparound sun glasses. If you do develop an allergy go to the doctor or the eye department of your hospital immediately. Our eyes are so precious but so delicate and sore eyes can also be extremely painful. A course of antibiotic eye drops will heal most eye problems but try not to wear eye make-up during the healing process. You will have to throw away any mascaras or eyeliners that you think may be infected and re sharpen eye pencils, otherwise you will just infect the other eye or re infect the first one.

If your eyes get sore regularly you may need more sleep but for an emergency pick me up pop on some eye pads (or slices of cucumber will do the trick) to bring down any puffiness and that tired look.

Not everybody can have perfect sight and most of us need reading glasses when we get older, so do have regular sight tests. What we eat and drink affects our eyes just as much as other parts of the body. So lay off the alcohol and eat regularly to keep your blood sugar up if you want to avoid blurred vision.

Spectacles are a big fashion accessory in today's world but if you do not fancy the idea, try contact lenses: there are lots of different types to suit most vision problems. You will have to look after your eyes even more carefully if you opt for lenses of course. I do not, for instance recommend doing what my delightful tennis partner OLWYN did when she dropped a lens on the all weather court at HOLMES PLACE/FULHAM, namely giving it a bit of lick and spit and bunging it back in her eye! Better by far to carry around a handbag sized bottle of "Refresh Contacts", available from good pharmacists, a self-explanatory product which is jolly useful as your eyes sometimes become tired and dry when wearing lenses. Another important tip if you are a lens wearer is not to get water on either your lenses or your lens case: water is as bad as spittle in this case.

Overleaf is a report on "eyes and eye care" from Mayfair opticians and contact lens practitioners JOHN DE CARLE (15 Brook's Mews, W1K 4DS, phone 020 7408 1208).

Laser eye surgery
The latest thing on the sight front is laser eye surgery which sounds miraculous but is it actually safe and does it hurt? I would be derelict in my duty if I did not report on this exciting new surgery so overleaf are all the details from one of the top laser eye surgery clinics in the UK ACCUVISION (42–48, New King's Road, SW6 4LS, phone 020 7736 2020 and Solihull).

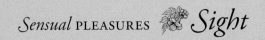

EYES AND EYE CARE

from John de Carle

Someone once said that next to life itself God's most precious gift to mankind was sight. This is so true yet how we take our sight for granted!

Fortunately, if we are born with healthy eyes and sight there is no maintenance required throughout our lifespan. There are however some useful exercises to do that will benefit the eye which will be mentioned later.

Like body types i.e. mesomorph, endomorph and ectomorph the eye can either become short sighted (myopic), long sighted (hyperopic) or remain normally sighted for most of our life span (emmetropic). Two other conditions play a part in the above three types and these are astigmatism and presbyopia. Astigmatism is where the surface of the eye is irregular (rugby ball or egg shaped) and causes a distorted picture. Presbyopia comes from Ancient Greek meaning "Old Eye". This is where the eye loses its ability to focus on near objects. This starts happening from birth at a very slow rate until we notice that we can no longer read small print around age 45–50 years. Hence the need for bifocals, varifocals or separate correction for distance and near vision.

How can we correct these errors (ametropias) in our vision?

Spectacles, contact lenses and laser surgery. For presbyopia or the ageing of the eye, varifocals or bifocals in either spectacle or contact lens forms can be used. Laser surgery is usually used to correct distance vision for either long or short sight but generally not for near vision problems.

Eyes usually reflect our general well-being and vitality. We so often remark on how well or unwell someone is by merely looking at their eyes. Eyes can also show happiness and sadness despite someone smiling. Some say the eyes are the windows to the heart and soul of an individual.

According to ancient Chinese medical thought, every sense organ is related to an organ, energy system and acupuncture meridian. In the case of the eye it is supposedly connected with the liver and its associated pathways. So if you want healthier looking eyes then look after your liver – less alcohol and rich, fatty foods. Start the day with hot water and lemon juice and if need be, some honey. This helps kick start the liver and should not be used symptomatically.

Some simple exercises for the eyes – such as looking near and far several times and gazing to all the compass angles several times including the obliques – all will benefit the ocular muscles and their circulation. Rotating eyes clockwise and counter clockwise can be done too. A more difficult exercise is to turn the head to the left simultaneously turning the eyes to the right. It may take a few attempts to get this co-ordinated.

Dr Bates (of "The Bates Method") advocated "Palming". Rubbing the palms together to generate warmth, place palms over closed eyes whilst supporting elbows on a table or desk, allow yourself to relax, subdue the mind and gaze into the black void for five minutes. This will revitalise the eyes and in some cases you may notice an improvement in the efficiency of perception – put it to the test. Remember, that the art of all this is in the practising of it!

Compresses can be used to good effect in increasing the circulation around the eye. Hot and cold but without extremes of temperature. Please note that if eyes are red and itchy as in the case of hay fever, then only cool to cold compresses may be used. With any inflammation, discharge or sensitivity to light, the eye must be examined professionally. In addition, routine visits to your optician are a must as many pathological conditions can be detected.

Cosmetic contact lenses can be used effectively either to enhance the natural colour of the eye or totally transform it depending upon the type of contact lens used. Severe corneal scarring from accidents can be masked or disguised with the use of contact lenses. Different eye colours in the same individual (heterochromic irides) can also be matched by wearing cosmetic contact lenses.

Symptomatic and palliative measures such as Optrex and other similar medicines that are vaso constrictive (shrink blood vessels and capillaries) may make the eye appear whiter but have no health benefit. Seek advice first before using any such eye drops as there may be an underlying infection or allergic cause.

Also here is all you need to know from an actual patient, FIONA who was thirty-five when she had her operation in 2004. FIONA wrote about her experience in detail (www.lasik-eyes.co.uk) and this is her account and opinion:

A patient's experience with Accuvision
"If you are thinking about having laser eye surgery, don't rush into it. Investigate several clinics and remember you don't have to commit to anything until you feel ready. When choosing a company, remember that you are purchasing eye

WAVEFRONT GUIDED LASIK AT ACCUVISION

from Accuvision

Laser Eye Treatment (LASIK) has become an everyday treatment for correcting vision, making it possible to throw away your contact lenses and glasses for good – just imagine the benefits! There are many clinics offering treatment and prices are becoming very competitive. However, you cannot put a price on your eyesight and it's very important to ensure you are making an informed choice about the surgery you are contemplating.

Accuvision are one of the UK's most technically advanced clinics being first to routinely carry out Wavefront guided technology considered to be the most advanced form of LASIK available today.

LASIK involves cutting a thin flap in your cornea and using a laser to smooth the surface to remove the "aberrations" that cause poor vision. After the procedure which lasts around one minute, the flap is replaced and your vision is immediately improved. Recovery takes around 24 hours and whilst the operation is a little uncomfortable, most people report no worse symptoms than "gritty" and dry eyes.

Like our fingerprints, each of our eyes is different and has its own unique shape and visual characteristics. Wavefront Guided Custom LASIK develops an individualised software treatment plan for each eye. Unlike the standard LASIK procedure which only corrects refractive errors (myopia, hyperopia and astigmatism) and routinely achieves 20/20 vision, Wavefront LASIK goes beyond just correcting refractive errors to actually improving visual capabilities so you may see better than you did with glasses or lenses before the procedure, hence improving your "Visual Acuity".

The visual system is actually capable of seeing 20/10 or better, that is letters twice as small as the 20/20 letters on an eye chart. Most people cannot see beyond 20/20 because of very subtle imperfections within their visual system. Using the Wavefront technology, it is possible to first map these subtle visual imperfections and then develop a laser treatment plan to correct them.

Accuvision believe that information is key and go to great lengths to ensure each patient is fully appraised of the procedure and potential risks, as well as the potential outcome post surgery, so that they can make their decision to proceed with knowledge and confidence. And it's important to remember that Accuvision's aim is not just to correct your vision – it's about improving the overall quality of your un-aided vision.

Although there are some people for whom LASIK is not suitable, with Accuvision's advanced technology, they are able to treat many people who have been turned down from having treatment at other clinics, including those with very high order aberrations (long and short sightedness) and also those with thin corneas.

You can visit Accuvision for a free, no obligation assessment to find out if you are suitable for surgery and also decide for yourself whether you are comfortable trusting them with your eyes.

surgery. Delicate eye surgery, not a winter sweater from a catalogue. You are only going to have this sort of thing done once, so chose wisely.

When I was researching LASIK, I came across several well-known clinics who were willing to offer me discounts if I introduced a friend or give me a 'buy one eye get one free' deal if I applied before a certain date. I walked away from all of them.

The scariest poster I saw announced 'big reductions on LASIK – end of season sale!' SALE?!… don't go there, please. Become as knowledgeable as you can on the subject so that you can quiz your chosen clinic as much as possible. Speak to people who have been treated by several different clinics and visit this web site: www.lasik-eye.co.uk

Once you have chosen your clinic, ask lots of questions. When you have an initial assessment, ask for copies of your test results and their surgeons' CVs – then go home and think about it some more.

Be aware of the risks and what you are committing yourself to. When I signed a consent form before surgery I accepted that there was a small chance that things may go wrong. I made that choice and accepted responsibility for my consent. This sounds scary, but it's the same with any surgical procedure. Your clinic can provide you with amazing technology but it is also your responsibility to look after yourself and follow the post-surgery guidelines.

Why I chose Accuvision
Small, friendly and highly knowledgeable company. No gimmicks or discounts. Not only was I treated as an individual but each of my eyes was too!

I requested copies of scans and the CVs of both surgeons and I was given all the information I wanted without question and without delay. The staff are very friendly and enthusiastic about their work. All my questions were listened to with respect and answered with patience in a language that I understood."

Sight 18

THE SENSUAL PLEASURES
OF SIGHT

CASTING our eyes at beautiful things is a truly sensual pleasure: for instance a bowl of pink tulips lit by the flames of a roaring log fire or maybe just looking into the flickering flames themselves. Of course those of us who have the money can buy beautiful "objets" to admire in their homes and beautiful jewellery to admire on their persons.

Things of beauty

Beautiful paintings can soothe our minds, inspire our souls and gladden our hearts. Whenever I have a bit of extra dosh (not often!) I toddle off to my sister-in-law Caroline's lovely art gallery, FARMILO-FIUMANO (27 Connaught Street, London, W2, phone 020 7402 6241) to find a painting to brighten the walls of our home. Or you could commission a portrait from talented PEREGRINE HEATHCOTE (07946 367 111, www.peregrineheathcote.com).

Jewellery is another thing entirely. There is so much good costume stuff around nowadays but sometimes it is reassuring to know that one is wearing The Real Thing, is it not? But the best sights are free: a beautiful sunset, a lush English garden in summer, a sparkling azure ocean.

Never forget that we have to be things of beauty ourselves who others, especially our husbands and boyfriends, will want to admire and covet. We can fill our homes with beautiful furniture, possessions and fresh flowers but we ourselves are the goddesses at the centres of our beautiful universes. If you have read the previous chapters carefully you will now know how to make the best of yourself through diet, fitness, beauty treatments and cosmetics. If you actually live with your man, however, he may not be too thrilled if your bedroom and bathroom are filled to overflowing with cosmetics, even though today's products are usually beautifully packaged. Plus, as I mentioned previously, men like to think that we ladies are natural beauties.

Permanent make-up

I have one more secret in my beauty arsenal which is particularly pertinent to ladies living with their gentlemen: semi-permanent make-up or "micro pigmentation" as the technique for applying it is called. This is eyeliner, eyebrow liner and lip liner that can be "tattooed" directly onto your skin so that your face always has some definition even when completely devoid of make-up. It is a totally brilliant idea that ensures you always look great in the bath, in the swimming pool, scuba diving or playing the most strenuous sport. The "s.p.m.u". usually lasts for about a year depending on which area it has been applied to and then you can have it re-applied. I myself have had both my mouth and my eyes outlined with this technique (my brows are already bushy-bushy!) and am completely hooked. It is so great to be able to get up in the morning and run out of the house with wide awake eyes and a luscious looking mouth without a scrap of the dreaded maquillage.

One of the leading practitioners of semi permanent make-up in the UK is DEBRA ROBSON-LAWRENCE (0845 230 2021, www.permanent-makeup.com) who is a renowned make-up artiste with years of experience and can often be seen on TV ("EXTREME MAKE OVERS", etc.). DEBRA says: *"Semi permanent make-up was first invented in the caveman era when our forbears used bones and plant matter to stain their skin. In its cosmetic form it was brought over from the States about 20 years ago.*

I developed my 'Facial Aesthetic Micro Enhancement' technique with my 'Liquid Perfection' pigments in the nineties. My style is very natural looking and softened down; for instance I can recreate individual hair strokes and effect a total eyebrow reconstruction. Originally I used to buy the pigments from the manufacturers but I noticed that the colours would change when

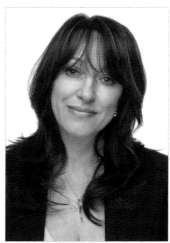

DEBRA ROBSON-LAWRENCE

combined with the actual skin. So I started working with the manufacturers and came up with my own range of natural, modern shades. I called the range 'Liquid Perfection' to give it a make-up rather than a tattooing feel. The pigments are made from iron oxide (a mineral) and stabilisers such as glycerine and alcohol and are completely safe, up to medical standard: in fact they can be used in hospitals.

Basically micro pigmentation is an advanced form of tattooing using different sized needles to create different effects on different areas. It is practically painless on the mouth and brows and just a little bit uncomfortable for some people around the eyes. Apart from the face I also use the technique on nipples and areolas (for ladies who have had cosmetic surgery where the incisions have been made in the areolas) or who have had breast reconstructions after mastectomies. It also works well to camouflage scars or small areas of Vitiligo.

My clients range in age from about 18 to 86! Micro pigmentation is particularly useful for more mature ladies whose lips have shrunk and/or have developed Alopecia of the brows and lashes as they have got older. I can outline around the lips to make them look fuller again, reproduce feathery hair for the brows and create simulated lashes in the outer corners of the eyes. It is also possible to do a full lip tint on the whole mouth and to dot in between the eyelashes with colours that complement the iris.

Ninety percent of women wear make-up every day: if they look better, they feel better and they feel that it helps them to attract partners, etc. You can still put make-up on over your semi permanent make-up but your features are already enhanced. I need two sessions with the client: the first application will be cautious and the second one four weeks later is for the 'fine tuning'. Your s.p.m.u. usually lasts about a year although if I apply it very softly or the client is out of doors in the elements a lot it may fade more quickly. In any case I like to redo it once a year to maintain a fresh look.

I can apply the s.p.m.u. to ladies who have had their lips and/or their eyes 'done' but I prefer to do the mouth before the lady has her 'filling' treatment if possible so that I can achieve the perfect outline and make the mouth symmetrical before it is injected. Of course you have to wait a certain amount of time after surgery before having micro pigmentation. If a lady has had a too severe brow lift and is looking too 'surprised' I can redraw the brow line lower down. Conversely I can open up the eyes by creating higher, more arched brows (withOUT Botox!) I can also fill in eyebrows after burning or ones that have been lasered off to remove a too heavily tattooed previous line. In other words I can provide the finishing touches to cosmetic surgery, improve bad work and 'reconstruct' brows after accident trauma. The technique really does not have any disadvantages.”

(In fact the only disadvantage I have ever found with s.p.m.u. was when I was filming a commercial in Holland in 2004 and the client wanted my face to appear completely make-up free. As you can imagine this was an horrific experience for moi and I was sick as a parrot when their make-up artiste dutifully concealed my gorgeous s.p.m.u.! But this was a totally extraordinary and hopefully unrepeatable "one off" experience which I hope fervently will never happen to you, dear readers.)

DEBRA also trains other ladies to apply "Liquid Perfection" and there are now micro pigmentation artistes nationwide. Another excellent London based practitioner is DAWN CRAGG (020 7224 2001). DAWN reports that she is busier than ever and that nipple tinting has now become very popular at her clinic!

PHOTO BY DAVID WILSON

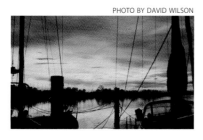
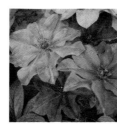
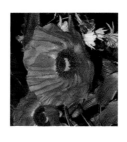
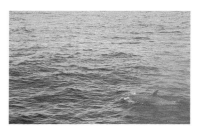

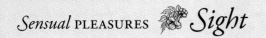

COLOUR ME CONFIDENT

from Veronique Henderson

Colour is integral to our lives. The colours you wear can have a profound effect on how you look and feel, as well as affecting your health and moods. Some colours will give you confidence and make you happy, while others can make you feel gloomy or drab.

In the right colours people will see **you** first – not what you are wearing. You will look and feel more healthy, confident, vibrant and even younger!

Choosing the right colours is all about finding harmony and balance with your skin, eye and hair colour. For example, women such as Catherine Zeta-Jones who have dark hair and dark eyes will suit strong rich shades such as chocolate brown, emerald green and burgundy. On the other hand, women like Cate Blanchett who have pale skin, naturally blonde hair, and blue or green eyes should stay clear of dark and rich colours which will make them look pale and tired. They should instead stick to lighter colours such as mint, sky blue, and pastel pinks.

Visiting an image consultant will help you understand which colours work best for you and ensure you are on your way to a co-ordinated wardrobe. Shopping will become easier and you will no longer be part of the majority of women who only wear 20% of what is hanging in their wardrobe.

Body Shapes

Wearing clothes in your colours is only the first step. It is just as important to wear clothes that compliment your build, body shape, proportions and personality. You also have to make sure that your are wearing the right style and fabrics to make the most of your assets.

An hourglass figure should enhance her curves. Wrap-around or cross-over tops and biased cut skirts can achieve this perfectly. In terms of fabric choose light to medium weights and textures such as cotton, jersey and silk.

If you have a straight body shape you may want to use some tricks to give the illusion of curves. Detail at the shoulders and bust line and again at the hips will achieve this, such as a full skirt combined with a bolero jacket.

For fuller figures, you want to create clean curves. Clothing lines need to be straight and fabrics should be soft and fluid. If you carry the majority of your weight on the lower half of your body, bring attention to the top half by adding details (i.e. prints, jewels) to your top half. The opposite rule applies if you carry the majority of your weight on the top half; choose tops and jackets with simple lines and deconstructed shapes.

If you are petite then the simpler the style the better; you don't want your clothes to be wearing you! Waist detail will cut your silhouette in half and will give a dwarfing effect. A sleek silhouette will succeed in elongating you as will any vertical detail. You may also prefer bias cuts or vertical seaming which draws the eye upwards acting as a subtle height enhancer.

Personality

Your personality is what dictates your style – your own interpretation of fashion and how you like to wear it.

For example:

The Natural

- Likes a relaxed, uncluttered look because comfort is of prime importance
- Has low maintenance hair and make-up

The Classic

- Likes to stay within safe combinations and avoids the latest fashion trends
- Finds it hard to dress down or mix and match their wardrobe

The Romantic

- Loves to get dressed up and indulge in long pampering sessions (long baths, manicures, etc.).
- Loves luxurious fabrics and details on clothing, wanting a totally feminine look

The Dramatic

- Loves fashion and wants to make a statement
- Likes to use colour in interesting ways and buys whatever accessories are in fashion

The Eurochic

- Understands what suits her, having tried lots of fashion trends
- Updates her wardrobe with accessories and different hair and make-up styles

What to wear

So that's your face but what about the rest of you? What to wear? What not to wear? Which clothes make you look best? The first thing you will need to know is which colours suit you and which do not. You can "get your colours done" and here the UK's top "colours" analyst, fashion expert VERONIQUE HENDERSON, of COLOUR ME BEAUTIFUL (020 7627 5211, www.cmb.co.uk, *Colour Me Confident* – Hamlyn, February 2006) gives you some fashion and colour tips on the page opposite.

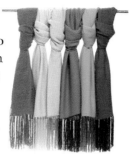

Body shapes

The second thing you need to take into account on the clothes front is your height and shape. You do not need fashion gurus TRINNY AND SUSANNAH to tell you this; just look in the mirror. Here are a few general tips:

- Shorter ladies should avoid patterns and outfits and accessories that cut them in half like large belts and three quarter length trousers and skirts.
- Larger girls should avoid white and light colours and, again, patterns and remember that black and navy are wonderfully slimming.
- If you feel you are too tall, wear flatties or low heels but hold yourself up and be proud of your height; no doubt you look like a goddess or a supermodel!

If you feel you are too thin, wear light colours and avoid black. The good news is that you can wear dayglo bright colours and patterns to your hearts' content.

Young girls can wear the shortest skirts and most outrageous designs as long as their legs and bod are reasonable.

More mature ladies should avoid the "mutton dressed as lamb" mistake and go for a more classy and classical look. If you are middle-aged (and I include myself here) or older you should strive for ageless beauty, timeless elegance

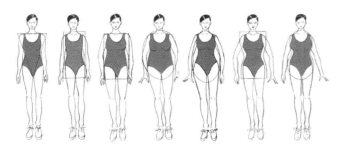

and all that. With the confidence of experience you will look superb in knee length little black dresses with loads of pearls and other jewellery, hats, gloves and the works. However if you are very mature you may prefer to cover your arms: think SOPHIA LOREN in her beautiful sheer black chiffon sleeves. Take a tip from JOAN COLLINS who manages to look amazingly sexy by just showing off her fabulous shoulders with the rest covered.

Fashion

Now if you have followed all the tips in the previous chapters your body should be as good as it will ever be so dress it with pride. Those of us with "loadsamoney" can toddle off to CHANEL, DIOR, VALENTINO, ARMANI and VERSACE to get kitted out. Haute Couture designs are always superbly flattering and made to measure garments will bring out the best in you. If you are lucky enough to have a perfect figure you can wear off the peg; a true goddess should look good in a sack, or at least a Greek tunic, but that would not be frightfully visually stimulating for our admirers!

Obviously we cannot all afford couture prices but in London there are a whole host of brilliant designers whose prices are affordable. My personal favourites are ROUBI EL ROUBI (9A Fitzgeorge Avenue, London, W14 0SY, phone 020 7602 9867, www.roubi.co.uk), ERIC WAY (020 7706 1358/07981 985 917, www.ericway.com), SAINT-HILL (20 Kinnerton Street, Belgravia, SW1, phone 020 7245 6778, www.saint-hillcouture.com) and PARVEEN (48 Dorset Street, London, W1, phone 020 7486 8480, www.parveen-couture.com), all of whose designs are flattering, feminine and unusual (we goddesses do not want to run into some other female wearing the same dress!) ROUBI EL ROUBI is the designer who (finally!) got me onto both the DAILY MAIL "Best Dressed" list and American TV with his stunning red "BAFTA" evening gown and who made busty JORDAN look classy and goddess like. ERIC WAY is the designer who made CHERIE BLAIR look sexy and KRISTIN DAVIES (Charlotte in *Sex and the City*) look both sexy and demure at once, not always an easy task. SAINT-HILL does great "floaties" and ASCOT outfits and PARVEEN also stocks beautiful jewellery and accessories in her shop so you can go for the total look.

One designer whose collections, especially her leathers and suedes, are always fun and feminine is ADELE BLOOM; phone 07976 728 880 for stockists of ADELE's unique "neo-romantic" and "champagne hippy" styles.

We all have our favourite little shops and one of *The Beach's* best treasure troves in Chelsea is BEYOND (285 Fulham Road, "The Beach", Chelsea, SW10 9PZ, phone 020 7351 2121) owned by chic fashion hound ESSAM GUENEDY. Here you can find unusual and classy day and evening outfits plus a brilliant selection of matching and toning accessories.

Do not despair if your frock budget is limited to the High Street: fashion is very affordable and accessible these days and there is something for everybody. Plus there are loads of Charity and second hand shops around where you can find real bargains. The best second hand designer shop in London is BERTIE GOLIGHTLY (48 Beauchamp Place, Knightsbridge, SW3 1NX, phone 020 7584 7270) which is chock full of gorgeous frox and accessories, including stunning hats if titfers take your fancy and you lead a posh enough life to wear them.

Accessories

One of the best kept secrets on the social circuit is SHEILA WARREN-HILL (020 8348 8282/07932 121196) who regularly holds first class designer sales at West End hotels or at her delightful house and garden in Highgate. SHEILA sells GUCCI, JOSEPH, YSL, PRADA et al clothes, MANOLO BLAHNIK shoes and gorgeous accessories at MARKS AND SPENCER prices. How does she do it? Like PRINCE CHARLES' alleged "fence", SHEILA sells "unwanted gifts" including whole wardrobes of clothes purchased from the sales of multi million pound estates. Bargains abound.

If you are getting married, congratulations! I suggest you visit London's RITVA WESTENIUS (Connaught Street, London, W2, phone 020 7060 7080) for something really stunning, meringue or otherwise, for this most important day in your life. If your daughter is getting married you should try PARVEEN COUTURE who specialise in both ready to wear and made to measure "Mother of the Bride" outfits.

Tiaras are an all important accessory if you are planning your nuptials or for "frightfully posh" do's. Freelance designer SHARIE-MARIE (020 7584 5948/ 07973 102 433) has an excellent selection and will also make to measure if required.

Accessories (or "hats and gloves and shoes and bags" as PATSY in *Absolutely Fabulous* calls them) make all the difference to your total look. It is worth investing in two really good daytime handbags (designer or fake as long as they are well made), dark for winter and light for summer, that will match everything. Shoes are great fun nowadays and you can pick up some cheap and cheerful ones on the High Street but, if you have got the dosh, I recommend treating yourself to JIMMY CHOO COUTURE (18 Connaught Street, London, W2, phone 020 7262 6888), MANOLO BLAHNIK (49 Old Church Street, Chelsea, SW3, phone 020 7352 3863) or TERRY DE HAVILLAND (07786 061 163). GINA (189 Sloane Street, Belgravia, SW1, phone 020 7235 2932) is another favourite for sexy sandals and mules.

Hats and gloves make all the difference to a smart outfit; gloves are very AUDREY HEPBURN and large, wide brimmed hats are sensationally flattering for all faces. The best gloves I have found are by CORNELIA JAMES, the glove manufacturer to THE QUEEN, which are stocked by the important department stores. For cheap and cheerful fun ones visit your local High Street.

Hats are not difficult to find in all the big stores but if you want something really special, try LOUIS MARIETTE (36A Sloane Gardens, London, SW1W 8DJ, phone 020 7730 3050, www.louismariette.com) for the prettiest cocktail hats in

WHY ONE NEEDS A STYLIST TO LOOK LIKE A GODDESS
from Lisa Maynard-Atem

Fashion has become so fast-paced that it is difficult to keep up with the latest trends. It is very easy to get lost in the latest look and the season's "must-have" item. A fashion stylist or image consultant can help to strip away all the jargon and work with you to develop a look that has longevity and ensures that, no matter the occasion, you always look like a goddess. Not only that, but having a stylist takes away the stress of having to trail around the shops, endlessly searching for the right clothes. Women have busy lives these days, with careers and children amongst everything else. There are not enough hours in the day to do everything. Being able to go to your wardrobe and pull out any outfit without the worry of how you will look in it, is a luxury that we all deserve.

Fashion stylists know all the tricks to making an outfit look perfect and can source those one-off pieces that no-one else will have or know where to find.

Why does one need a stylist to look like a goddess? My answer to that is simple – to ensure that you always look fabulous… even if you are just popping out to the corner shop!

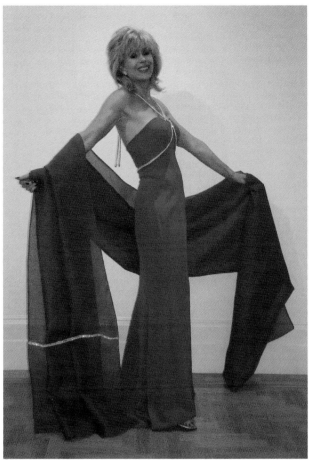

© GABOR SCOTT   SALLY WEARING ROUBI EL ROUBI BAFTA DRESS AND SHAWL

town and DEIDA ACERO (deida@deidahats.com) for the most divine special occasion titfers you will ever see.

Stylists

If you still have trouble putting yourself together fashion wise you can always hire a stylist. This may well prove a good investment and will save you a great deal of time and trouble, not to mention money spent on "mistakes". Stylist LISA MAYNARD-ATEM's report is opposite (07745 544 418, enquiries@stylisa.com, www.stylisa.com)

Your home is an extension of yourself and should always look attractive and welcoming. If you cannot afford a decorator learn to paint the walls yourself; it is not that difficult. Pastel colours are easiest to live with on your walls: pale green is very soothing, pale pink gives a warmer glow than white or magnolia and pale yellow is very cheerful whereas too much pale blue can look cold. You can liven up your rooms with brighter colours; for instance everyone loves the shocking pink silk KELLY HOPPEN curtains in the

"adults' living room" at our home. They look really expensive but actually came from THE CURTAIN EXCHANGE (131 Stevendale Road, Fulham, SW6, phone 020 7731 8316), a wonderful second hand curtain shop.

A little bit of disarray in a home makes it look lived in and is not unattractive but "cleanliness is next to Godliness", health goddesses, so get thee going with the feather duster! Remember, though, the more knick knacks you have, the longer you will take to dust them. If, like me, you are not naturally domesticated employ a really good cleaner as often as possible. I use a professional cleaning company called KLEANKEEPERS (Spaces Business Centre, 35A Ingate Place, London, SW11 3NS, phone 020 7978 2004, www.kleankeepers.co.uk) who keep our home looking suitably pleasing to the eye and save me from having a nervous breakdown. If, however, you prefer to do your own cleaning either for personal or economical reasons, it will help you to stay fit; just don't forget to wear your MARIGOLDS on your pampered, goddess like hands.

Once you and your home are looking sensually pleasurable, think about the food you are going to serve. Presentation is all important: a meal that looks, as well as tastes and smells, delicious can tempt even the faddiest eater and somehow seems more filling to a dieter because your eyes are satisfied as well as your stomach.

Three course menu – presentation

ANTON MOSIMANN, OBE is the famous Swiss born chef who garnered two (GUIDE) MICHELIN stars for London's DORCHESTER HOTEL. In 1988 he opened MOSIMANN'S (Mosimann's Private Dining Club, 11B, West Halkin Street, Belgravia, SW1X 8JL, phone 020 7235 9625, www.mosimann.com), his exclusive dining club in Belgravia, membership of which is coveted and which has a Royal warrant. (Yes, the great ANTON cooks for Royalty on a regular basis, including for PRINCE CHARLES and THE DUKE OF EDINBURGH!) MOSIMANN's superb cookery shows and books have made him a huge TV and media star and in 1996 he set up the MOSIMANN ACADEMY in order to share his knowledge of and passion for cooking. In 1985 he created "Cuisine Naturelle", a new and healthy style of cooking which eschews the use of fat and alcohol. It goes without saying that MOSIMANN's presentation is second to none. For these best of reasons I asked the delightful ANTON to create a healthy nutritious three course meal which would look every bit as good as it tasted and here it is on the next page.

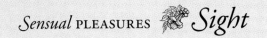

THREE COURSE MENU – PRESENTATION
from Anton Mosimann, Mosimann's Private Dining Club

Course one: Starter
Marinated salmon with Cornish crabmeat   Serves 4

MARINADE
20 g coriander seeds
150 g sea salt
150 g castor sugar
20 g white peppercorns
20 g star anise
2 sticks lemon grass
zest of 2 lemons
Blend ingredients roughly in a food processor.

SALMON
500 g salmon fillet, skin on
Spread the above mixture all over the salmon. Marinate for 24 hours. Wash the marinade off, skin the salmon and remove the brown fat. Slice the salmon in thin slices and arrange on a plate in a 5½ inch ring. Keep the ring on the plate.

CRABMEAT
100 g picked white crabmeat
5 g sliced chives
12 leaves coriander
20 g finely sliced spring onions
12 pieces pickled ginger
Sprinkle the crabmeat evenly over the salmon. Garnish with the rest of the ingredients and remove the ring.

LEMON DRESSING
juice of 4 lemons
50 g castor sugar
a little arrowroot
100 ml olive oil
100 ml sunflower oil
20 ml light soya sauce
Bring the lemon juice and the sugar to the boil; combine arrowroot and soya sauce, thicken lemon juice to sauce consistency. Whisk in oil slowly. Clean plate and drizzle the dressing over the top of the salmon and crab

Course two: Main course
Poached chicken breast stuffed with baby leeks and trompette mushrooms, tomato and herb dressing   Serves 4

POACHED CHICKEN
4 maize-fed chicken breasts, with bone trimmed and cleaned
Remove skin from breasts. Place them on a chopping board and using a knife butterfly each breast, cover with cling film and gently flatten with a rolling pin.
8 baby leeks
Blanch leeks in boiling salted water until just tender, drain, cool in ice water and set aside.
100 g fresh or 10 g dried trompette mushrooms
If using fresh mushrooms, clean them and tear in half. If using dried, soak mushrooms in warm water for ten minutes, tear them in half and wash well to remove dirt and sand. Drain well.

TO PREPARE THE CHICKEN
Salt and pepper
Chicken stock for poaching
Spread cling film on cutting board. Sprinkle with salt and pepper. Spread the breast on the cling film and season with salt and pepper. Place two leeks and some mushrooms along the centre and roll up. Then roll the breast with the cling film to a sausage, twist both ends and make a knot. Repeat with other three chicken breasts. Poach for 10–12 minutes in chicken stock. When ready remove from stock and keep warm.

TOMATO AND HERB DRESSING
3 plum tomatoes
100 ml olive oil
70 ml reduced chicken stock
30 ml sherry vinegar
10 ml French mustard
salt and pepper
2 tbsp finely chopped chives
2 tbsp finely chopped chervil
1.5 tsp finely chopped dill
While chicken is poaching, blanch the tomatoes in boiling water for approx ten seconds, remove and drop into cold water. Remove skin, cut in quarters and remove seeds and cut into dice. Whisk together the olive oil, vinegar, reduced chicken stock and mustard. Season to taste and set aside.
Just before serving gently warm the dressing in a small pan and add the herbs and tomatoes.

TO SERVE
Remove the cling film from the chicken breast and cut in two at an angle. Place into the centre of individual plates and drizzle over some of the tomato dressing. Serve with market vegetables.

Course three: Dessert
Lavender and vanilla pannacotta   Serves 4

THE PANNACOTTA
450 ml double cream
100 ml milk
50 g castor sugar
2 vanilla pods
1 tbsp lavender flowers – chopped
bronzed gelatine leaves
Bring the milk, sugar, vanilla pods and lavender to the boil, then remove from heat and allow to infuse for 15 minutes.
Add the pre-soaked gelatine leaves to the milk mixture, stirring until dissolved.
Strain into a different bowl and put into the fridge allowing the mixture to cool.
When the mixture is thickened and coats back of spoon pour into the required moulds. Allow to set in the fridge for about 2–3 hours then demould, by running hot water over the bottom to loosen.
Then serve and decorate with seasonal fruits and berries.

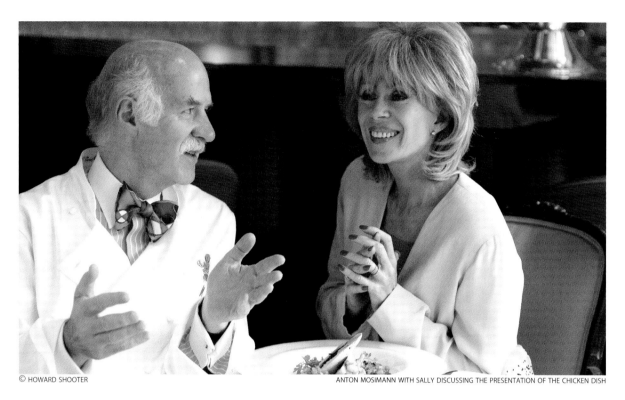

© HOWARD SHOOTER   ANTON MOSIMANN WITH SALLY DISCUSSING THE PRESENTATION OF THE CHICKEN DISH

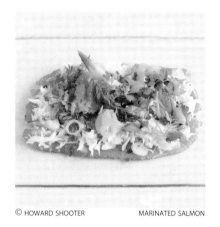

© HOWARD SHOOTER   MARINATED SALMON

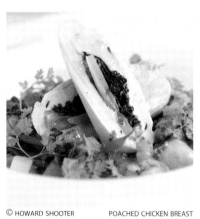

© HOWARD SHOOTER   POACHED CHICKEN BREAST

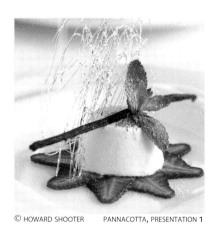

© HOWARD SHOOTER   PANNACOTTA, PRESENTATION 1

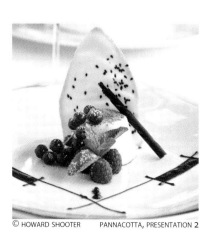

© HOWARD SHOOTER   PANNACOTTA, PRESENTATION 2

Hearing 19 & Sound

EAR CARE
REMEDIES & METHODS

.

Y ex, legendary record producer STEVE ROWLAND (from whom we will hear in the next chapter) always used to say "these are ears, not garbage pails", meaning "do not insult me with words and sounds I do not want to hear". Fair enough but we all want to hear sensually pleasurable words and sounds and therefore the first step is to look after our ears properly. Our ears affect our balance as well as our hearing so if you have any sort of ear problem whatsoever you must go to the doctor or to an ear, nose and throat specialist immediately. In some cases you may need to have your ears syringed which is not a particularly pleasurable experience but will improve your hearing. If you have a serious hearing problem you may need a hearing aid but, never fear, they are really tiny and discreet these days.

HOT GOSSIP UK's consultant GP, DR RICHARD HART (020 8952 5536) says "when you are washing your face and neck do be careful not to get any soap and water inside your ears. Never try to clean inside your ears with your finger or a cotton bud as some people do, just clean the outsides of the ears". For those of you who use ear plugs for sleeping, you must be especially careful. Only use wax plugs (BOOTS' "Muffles" are the best I have found) and never push them in too far. If you do push a plug (or anything) too far inside your ear as I once did, lie flat on the bad ear and pour a little warmed oil into the other ear: the plug or object will pop out quite soon.

The latest "technology" for ear health is actually an ancient Native Indian remedy involving HOPI and essential oil ear candles. You just lie down while a second person puts the candle into your ear and lights the top of it; it is called an "Indian Relaxation Ceremony" which calms the mind and soothes the head as well as the ears. As the candle burns down to the safety filter you will hear a gentle crackling sound. When the candle is removed you will see that all the excess wax and dried skin which was present in your ear has been collected in the filter and can now be binned. The ritual is very relaxing as well as deep cleansing for your ears and aids your breathing and sense of smell as well as your hearing, whilst also ridding you of headaches if you are a sufferer. HOPI ear candles can be ordered from the Internet at: www.sortlifeout.co.uk and are quite reasonable. However before sticking anything into your delicate ears you should know more about it and do read all the HOPI information and instructions carefully before beginning the "ceremony".

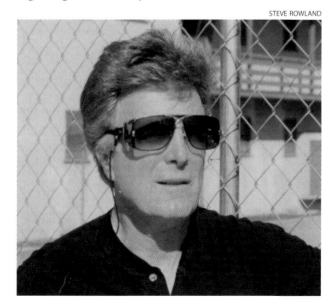

STEVE ROWLAND

Hearing 20 & Sound

SOUND & MUSIC

HEARING is the most immediate of the senses; apparently what we hear affects us even faster than what we see. Sound and music add audio "colour" to our lives. Imagine a film or television show without its music: the "scoring" sets the scene and tells our senses what to expect and what we should feel in that scene. We can "score" our lives with music: for instance factories use up tempo music to encourage their staff to work faster and we can make ourselves more dynamic by playing fast pop music while we are exercising or doing the housework. Music is "the food of love" and uplifts our souls. Playing romantic music will put you and your loved one (or the one you want to hit on!) in the mood for lurrrve any time, any place, anywhere. Personally I favour the lush strings of ANDREW LLOYD-WEBBER to uplift my soul especially if I am driving in the city when most of us are likely to be just a touch crabby! Beautiful classical music is also very uplifting and can soothe our spirits and helps us to relax. STRAUSS waltzes will make anyone feel like a goddess, especially *Also Sprach Zarathustra*, more popularly known as the theme tune from the classic film *2001*.

Favourite music

Here are some suggestions for using sensually pleasurable and stimulating music in different areas of our lives. Firstly from KARDY LAGUDA, choreographer and dance-aerobiciser extraordinaire on music to work out to:

"I feel that you can use the following tracks for a good aerobic workout:

Disco Tracks
1. *Blame it on the Boogie (Club Mix) – The Jacksons*
2. *September 99 – Earth Wind & Fire (Phats and smalls Remix)*

Other
1. *California Dreaming – Royal Gigolos*
2. *Hi Energy 2004 – Evelyn Thomas*
3. *Flashdance – Deep Dish (R. Rincon Remix)"*

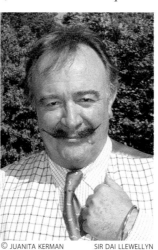

© JUANITA KERMAN   SIR DAI LLEWELLYN

Now here is SIR DAI LLEWELLYN, the original "seducer of the valleys," on music for seduction:

"I think the old albums are the best ones; 'Only You' by THE PLATTERS, 'True Love' by BING CROSBY AND GRACE KELLY, 'Smoke Gets In Your Eyes' by BRYAN FERRY, 'THE ROCKY HORROR SHOW' soundtrack featuring SUSAN SARANDON singing 'I Want To Be Dirty' and SHANIA TWAIN's 'That Don't Impress Me Much'".

On the romantic front most people favour the music of blind artiste ANDREA BOCACCIO whose sense of hearing has undoubtedly been sharpened by sadly having one less sense. Personally I find LLOYD-WEBBER's "Phantom of the Opera" incredibly romantic but guys do not always agree with me!

Listening to music will give your life and everything in it an extra dimension. Record producer STEVE ROWLAND told me his favourite music to live by is:

- *"EVA CASSIDY 'Songbird'. She is one of the greatest voices of her generation. Fantastic. She died of cancer in her early thirties.*
- *BOB MARLEY and THE WAILERS 'Legend'. This is a compilation of his greatest hits, including 'Jamming', 'Exodus', 'No Woman No Cry' and many more.*
- *FRANK SINATRA with the RED NORVO QUINTENT 'Live in Australia, 1959'. 19 of his greatest hits – live in concert. He's never sounded better.*
- *BUENA VISTA SOCIAL CLUB Cuba's greatest jazz musicians. There was a film documentary made about this group of musicians. They are considered some of the best in the world. Castro suppressed their music for years by not allowing it to be heard outside of Cuba.*
- *RAY CHARLES. He's a true musical genius. He has inspired so many of today's top singers and musicians. I am one of them. Every album he's ever made has been a masterpiece."*

STEVE reckons his favourite music to drive to is ZZ TOP, BARRY WHITE, TAMMIE WYNETTE and NORA JONES whereas I find BUDDY HOLLY and S CLUB JUNIORS calm my nerves at the wheel (well, it takes all types!) Basically all of our lives need a bit of mood enhancing sometimes and the way to do it is with music, not with drugs, pills and alcohol.

Different sounds have different connotations: the drone of a jet or the vroom of an outboard motor always make me think of sensually pleasurable summers on THE COTE D'AZUR but are hard to recreate in one's own home. There are various audio tapes you can buy with suitably soothing sounds on them like waves gently lapping on the shore which are perfect for relaxation, stress relief and insomnia. One of the best for "relieving anxiety for women" is SAMANTHA WILSON's "Stress Soother" tape, available from The Clinic, 56 Harley House, Marylebone Road, London, NW1, phone 020 7486 4115.

Meditation

The subject of stress leads me to meditation which in itself is an important subject because we all want our minds to be every bit as healthy as our bodies. Harley Street meditation expert RAHAT AFZAL SHEIKH, MBIH, EHP, NLP (RELAXATION RESPONSE MEDICAL CENTRE, 1 Harley Street, London W1G 9QA, phone 020 7291 4450, www.positivepeace.co.uk and HB HEALTH, 12 Beauchamp Place, London SW3, phone 020 7838 0765, www.hbhealthonline.com) who has herself to have the most blissfully soothing voice, told me:

MEDITATION
from Rahat Afzal Sheikh

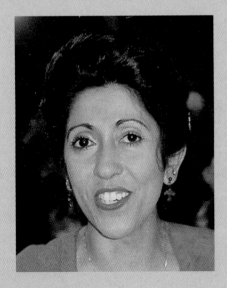

A visit to the Relaxation Response and Meditation Centre is an educational journey where you learn that well being is a mental, physical, emotional and spiritually balanced state. You learn to gain understanding of your breathing and the inner power and to know you can change old and negative patterns. This is a key to learning which is worth its weight in gold. Stepping away from recurring negative patterns in relationships, anger, confusion, illness, insecurity, addictions and fear.

This education changes you into a balanced person who can attract people and circumstances into your life and enhance positive prosperity.

The Relaxation Response Technique is a process of meditation designed to create an altered state of consciousness characterised by a separation of mind, body and all the inner senses to see, feel, smell, touch, hear and think clearly. This at the same time with repetition increases the feeling of oneness, increased self-understanding, acceptance of relationships and the set of circumstances in the personal world around you. Achieve inner peace and tranquillity.

If you can see a bottle with muddy water – imagine drop by drop of clear water in it, eventually achieving absolute clarity as you see it happening naturally. This technique is designed through meditation and its rules show you how to feel your inner depths.

Meditation has claimed to give self-awareness and balanced relationships towards others. Understanding yourself more clearly and thereby achieving greater self-esteem and growth. Decreasing stress, anxiety and even improved performance in everything personally, at work and in sports.

Meditation method

There is no single "right" way to create a meditation state. Methods developed over the years range from sitting quietly with closed eyes to the ecstatic dancing of Sufi "whirling dervishes". So procedures involve opening up attention by calmly pausing; others use a focusing method – a word, an object or a sound.

Unique Relaxation Response and Meditation

Tried, tested and trusted method.

Method – Sufi Meditation

Engage all your natural senses to oneness and a peacefully balanced state. Naturally over time you reach a point of balance and further connection to your spiritual senses and increase a real awareness of your life just by letting go. Relax and discover you have qualities and abilities within you to feel empowered. Use your own keys to success.

Sit in a comfortable chair, breathe in deeply and think the word "relax". Now slowly breathe all the way out. Think the word "relax". Repeat this ten times.

- Now imagine a fruit basket with lots of different fruit in it
- Choose a piece of fruit
- Hold it in your hands. (Think the word "relax")
- Feel the texture.
- Touch it. (Think the word "relax")
- Peel the fruit and slice it
- Smell the fruit and taste it
- Let the energy trickle down your throat. (Think the word "relax")
- How nature has the balance in the fruit – the colour, the smell, the taste, the energy. You also have this balance in you to think clearly, feel at ease, make choices and decisions that bring positive benefits in your life
- Do your deep breathing
- Think the word "RELAX"

Repeat above exercise and link to your inner senses

As simple as it appears, it has a very powerful promise to relax to a level that is just right for you. Each one of us at some point in our lives has one or more of our senses in self preservation. This simple technique allows you to naturally relax and discover it is okay to see, feel, understand and let go. Make your mind your best friend. (Switch it off for a moment). If we are aware of our physical stress we release it and maintain

a quality of life. Further guided meditations include other levels and the key to enlightenment.

Effects of Relaxation Deepen Meditation Technique

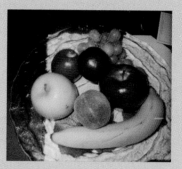

During a typical meditation session respiration, heart rate, muscle tension, blood pressure and oxygen consumption decrease. Meditators commonly report feeling deep relaxation and inner peace. They may also experience significant decreases in such problems as general anxiety, high blood pressure, alcoholism, drug addition, insomnia and all other stress related problems. Anger, dysfunctional relationships, sexual and emotional disturbances. Meditators' scores in personality tests indicate increases in general health, self esteem and social openness (Shapiro & Giber 1978).

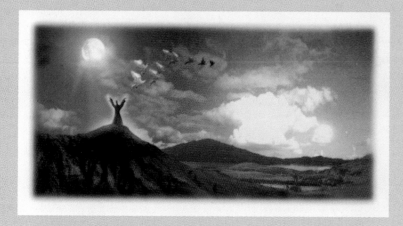

The soul of the Universe speaks to us. Everything and everyone naturally reveals their own purpose. Open up the link to your inner senses and you are able to contact the voice of everything. Every day is luminous as we seek the treasure reserved for us.

© 1997 Rahat Sheikh

Snoring

Sadly some sounds are not as sweet as others. Snoring can be the bane of one's existence and is something that is very hard to cure. If your partner snores you may have to resort to earplugs (BOOTS' "Muffles" wax ones are the best, as I mentioned earlier) but make sure you have regular sessions with your HOPI ear candles in case any plug wax gets into your ear. If you yourself are the snorer that is bad luck and not particularly goddess like but the problem is not insuperable. This is what VALERIE AUSTIN, author of *Self Hypnosis* told me about how to deal with this sensually unpleasurable affliction.

"*It is sometimes difficult to cure people of snoring even with hypnosis, because the causes are varied and are usually rooted in a physical problem of some kind, but of course not always. However, there is hope for those who have to sleep near someone who snores.*

For people who sleep near people who snore:
It is because you love being so alive and wide awake during the day that you also adore the rejuvenation and bliss of tranquil, deep sleep during the night… in this sleep, your body does marvellous things… it looks after itself and it looks after you… it just carries on with its many functions without you even having to be aware of it in any way.

In this sleep your subconscious reigns… you travel far in your dreams, seeing your future in the best possible light… all your plans and aspirations are seeded here… at night, you love to sleep… your desire to sleep is so profound that should you ever hear sound, it will only act as a trigger for you to dream… the more noises you hear, the better you sleep… since these will form the gentle pleasant background noises within your wondrous dreams.

Best of all… should you have the good fortune to sleep near someone who snores, his or her breathing rhythm immediately causes you to breathe more slowly and deeply… just like the slow ticking of a grandfather clock… tick… tock… tick… tock… the louder the snore, the deeper you sleep.

The sound of snoring will always bring a feeling of safety and calm, followed by a most profound sleep… with dreams of vibrant health… wealth and happiness… and, what's more, you always wake up smiling!

On one of my residential courses early in the 90s one of the students snored very, very loudly. The person sharing the room, Pierre, couldn't sleep at all.

The next day I asked Pierre to write a script and use it in self-hypnosis. He did this and the next morning he happily reported that he had slept so much better. He said that he was lucky that his roommate hadn't snored. I had passed the room late at night and the loudest snoring noises were coming from it. The suggestion worked and he never heard the snoring for the rest of the week."

Getting dead drunk will often make you snore so avoid it, ladies: it simply is not goddess like!

Insomnia

Snoring and insomnia do not necessarily go together and insomnia is actually much more serious and potentially detrimental to your health. If your problem is chronic you must visit the doctor but, in the long run, sleeping pills and Valium are bad for you and you must find a permanent and healthy solution. Insomnia can affect anyone at any time especially if you are stressed or during hormonal periods in your life such as puberty, pregnancy and menopause. If you have tried herbal remedies, Horlicks, hot baths with Radox and counting sheep to no avail the time may have come for you to try hypnotherapy. Opposite VALERIE AUSTIN explains hypnotherapy for this ticklish problem.

I myself have suffered from insomnia and found it extremely debilitating but was successfully treated by VALERIE. Do not wait around for the problem to go away by itself; get professional help immediately before you become totally exhausted and lose your quality of life.

VALERIE AUSTIN

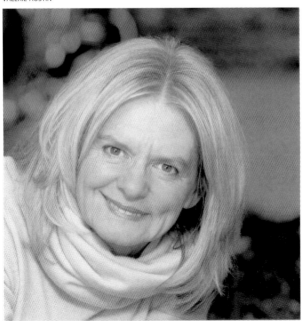

HYPNOTHERAPY FOR INSOMNIA

from Valerie Austin

What is a caught condition? It could have started from your partner snoring, work stress, etc. or new noises that keep you awake creating the bad "habit" of insomnia. You may have changed partners but still suffer from bouts of insomnia – this could simply be habit which is corrected by suggestions in trance – self-hypnosis.

What is a trauma condition? When something happens in childhood that is traumatic and stops you from sleeping. Then you may sleep normally until later in life when you have a similar experience that sets it off again. You may think you know when it started, for example only a few years ago when you were changing your job or lost your partner, but in fact it goes much further into your past buried safely in your subconscious.

The trauma may have been serious when you were a child but not so now – just one of the many traumas we have when we are children simply growing up. It doesn't have to be frightening to us now.

Hypnosis is the tool to bring the information to the surface so it can be resolved – the result is peaceful sleep.

This trauma based insomnia problem generally needs a professional therapist to get to the root of the problem. You also need to check that the hypnotherapist you choose is a skilled regressional therapist. Not all hypnotherapists use regression and some use it seldom so they are not very skilled. When I teach my courses for a career in hypnotherapy I teach the skill of regression which ensures a very high success rate.

However, whichever type of insomnia you may have no harm can be done in trying the self-help first. It gives you a tool to work with yourself and also saves the expense of a therapist if you can cure yourself.

My advice as a specialist in hypnotherapy is that if you find self-hypnosis is not working for you then look for an experienced regression therapist. It is a bit like going to the DIY store to save money – some people find it much easier than others because they are more committed.

A Basic Relaxation Exercise:

The simple words below or the long progressive induction mentioned earlier can be used to ease you into a trance followed by a suggestion for insomnia or weight or whichever problem you wish to deal with. You can tape yourself and play it back or get a friend or relation to read it slowly to you. Make sure the person you choose is not the type to giggle but will take it seriously.

The Relaxer

This type of exercise helps you to control tension. Practise it once a day for three weeks. It gives you a chance to establish the habit of relaxing. Then practice it once a week for a short time. Later, a booster every now and then will suffice.

When you feel comfortable with it add the suggestion for insomnia. Opposite, I have included a suggestion if you are the partner of a person who snores. This has helped many people to no longer have sleepless nights and even saved marriages.

Close your eyes and take a deep breath in…allow yourself to exhale fully and completely…making sure you get the last air out of your lungs…breathe in again…as you inhale, allow yourself to see number "1" in your mind's eye…at the same time focus your mind on your inhalation…hold your breath for approximately 3 seconds and then exhale…as you breathe the air out fully and completely…mentally say to yourself "2" and visualise the number "2" in your mind's eye…breathe in again…and mentally visualise the number "3"…hold your breath for 3 seconds…and then exhale fully and completely…while mentally visualising and saying "4"…inhale "5" and exhale again saying "6"…always remembering to visualise the number and to focus your mind on your breathing…inhale and see the number "7"…and exhale counting "8"…then "9"…and now "10".

Repeat the full sequence once again, keeping your eyes closed. Picture yourself resting comfortably. Visualise it in your mind's eye…you are so relaxed.

Count backwards from ten to one slowly, easily and more rhythmically to bring yourself out of the relaxation.

Hypnosis induction that you can tape and then play back

Suggestion for insomnia: Choose a chair that is very comfortable and start to use visualisation to put you into a light trance.

Insomnia: You find you sleep soundly and peacefully for the length of time you require – your dreams are pleasant.

You can imagine yourself calm and relaxed and comfortable relaxing deeply with each breath. You picture yourself asleep and your chest moving up and down. As soon as you close your eyes when you put your head on the pillow you feel drowsy and slip into sleep very quickly.

If you want to mull over the day's events before you go to sleep the time will seem to pass far more quickly than usual and you find ways to put this time to constructive use. The sleep you have is so deep and relaxing that you awake at the correct time – refreshed and relaxed and ready to begin a new day. When you have less time than usual to sleep, the sleep you have is more effective… Every hour seems like two hours and you wake up refreshed.

You sleep soundly, peacefully for the time required and you are drowsy and relaxed and as soon as you put your head on your pillow you fall asleep immediately.

Hearing & Sound

21

VOICES

WHAT do *you* sound like? Does your voice give listeners the sensual pleasure of a purring pussycat or does it jangle the nerves like a screech owl? We all know the story of how silent screen idol RUDOLPH VALENTINO's career was ruined when the "talkies" arrived because his weedy reedy voice did not match up to his smouldering good looks. On the other hand we have modern actress JOANNA LUMLEY whose gorgeously silky smooth and caressing voice can sell a hundred products and wow the gentlemen long distance. She is one "English Rose" beauty whose voice actually sounds every bit as inviting as her face and figure.

In this modern day and age when so much business is done on the phone a "good" voice is all important. On the romantic front you can woo your lover vocally and "telephone sex" has never been more popular! People have fallen in love with voices alone so make sure yours is as appealing as it can be. Of course the rest of you needs to meet up to the exacting standards of your goddess like voice but by this point in my book you should know how to look your best as well as sound your best at all times.

If you are less than confident about your voice you may need to visit a speech therapist. If it is good enough for PRINCESS DIANA, BARONESS THATCHER and DAVID BECKHAM then it is good enough for us. Just remember that softer, lower voices are always more attractive than high, strident ones and that a nasal quality is very off putting. There may be some medical reason why you speak through your nose and if your HOPI ear candles have not cleared your nose, get your sinuses checked at the doctor's. If you speak through your nose for other reasons then the bad habit can be unlearnt with a vocal therapist.

Regional accents are quite acceptable nowadays so do not be embarrassed if you do not speak with a cut glass Oxford English accent. If people really cannot understand what you are saying then you will need elocution lessons but a little bit of your origins is actually very appealing. For instance a trace of Welsh, light Morningside Scottish or a gentle West Country burr can give an interesting quality to your speech. If you are foreign, do retain your exotic French, Latin or Scandinavian lilt and remember how keen guys are on Southern belle drawlers like JERRY HALL, another gal whose sexy voice lives up to her stunning appearance.

Even a Cockney or South London accent can be appealing if the voice itself is pretty. DENISE VAN OUTEN is very goddess like, for instance. But the tone and pitch of your voice is more important than the accent. Vocal coach TESSA WOOD, AGSM, PGDVS-CSSD/Dip Ed (TessaRossWood@aol.com) says:

Educating the voice

"Elocution deals with what happens in the mouth and is purely concerned with accent. Voice training deals with the whole body and is not necessarily about removing an accent – although this can be done on request.

The foundation for a good voice comes from two main things: the way you breathe and the way you stand, sit or move around – your physical alignment. Because a good voice involves your whole body, it is essential the body work in harmony. If, for example, you tend to slump or rest on one leg, placing your body out of alignment, you will struggle to access the breath you need.

Simply by adjusting your alignment by a few millimetres, you are able to breathe more effectively and release the voice more freely. Don't take my word for it, try it.

Either sitting or standing, slump in your spine and try to breathe to the lowest part of your lungs and say, 'Friends, Romans, countrymen, lend me your ears'. Then try speaking it sitting up or standing tall. Breathe to the lowest part of your lungs before speaking. Did you notice any difference? It can take a little while, but with practice you can give your voice more gravitas and a much more connected and compelling quality.

Of course, there are other things to consider in finding your free voice: how much space you make in your mouth, how much variety in pitch and tone you use. You also need to make friends with your tongue! But there are a range of exercises which are fun to do and very effective if performed regularly.

Some people find they can get help from books such as Patsy Rodenburg's The Right To Speak, or Cicely Berry's Your Voice and How to Use It, but for better and often quicker results, a good voice class like those offered at London's 'City Lit' or comparable will do the trick.

Voice – does it matter?

Picture, in your mind's eye, an aspiring professional – man or woman, anyone from an actor or advertising executive to a stockbroker or scientist.

TESSA ROSS WOOD

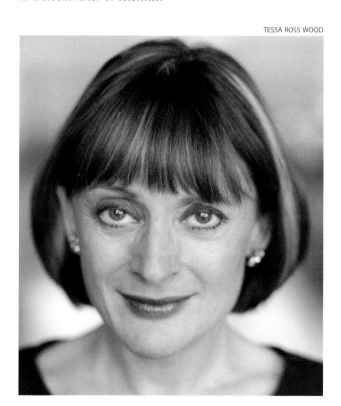

Keep them in your mind's eye and see them as immaculately dressed – Armani, Joseph – or anything you like. Imagine the hair, accessories – all expensive and every detail carefully planned. The image should speak of confidence and success.

Now imagine that same person preparing to address a meeting or about to give a presentation. See them looking wonderful as they move into position to start. Then imagine them speaking. They open their mouth, and a thin, whiney voice is emitted – or perhaps one that is shrill and rasping, or even one so tiny, you have to strain to hear. What does that do to the immaculate image in front of you?

Some people are able to listen selectively and edit out any negative vocal qualities. We do it all the time with certain politicians and celebrities! But it can place the speaker at a disadvantage and detract from what they are trying to say.

Why is it, do you suppose, that the average professional spares no time or expense on their visual persona but neglects the most important aspect of their personal presentation: voice? The part that communicates your inner thoughts so directly to the outside world. Is it because it doesn't matter? I don't think so.

One of the main reasons is that rather like health people tend to take it for granted until something goes wrong. But another reason is that most people don't realise how relatively easy it is to make changes – and once acquired, these changes can last a lifetime.

What is a 'good voice'? A good voice is one that is free, resonant, clear and compelling. It is not one that has been 'elocuted' only.

Back to training your voice: of course group classes are not tailor made to the individual, as there can be 20 or more others, each with vocal idiosyncrasies. For bespoke one-to-one sessions you need a good private voice coach. But a word of warning here. In our de-regularised world, there are a number of people who set themselves up as voice gurus who have no recognised qualifications. To protect your voice from damage or just ineffective teaching, you should try to find someone with a specialist diploma or MA like that granted from The Central School of Speech and Drama.

If you're not sure whether or not someone is recognised, you can call Central on 020 7722 8183. Also the British Voice Association (BVA) – 020 7713 0064 is a wonderful source of information that also has a comprehensive website (www.british-voice-association.com).

You may not end up sounding like DAME JUDI but with a little work on your part you will almost certainly sound clearer, stronger and a more compelling version of yourself.

Good luck!"

Touch

22

STROKING & MASSAGE

Some people think that touch is the most important of the five senses. Certainly it is the most comforting with hugs, kisses, handholding and back stroking on the agenda and not just for babies and the elderly! Then there is "The Joy of Sex" to quote DR ALEX COMFORT, an aptly named practitioner.

A recent SUNDAY TIMES report extolled the virtues of back stroking for women telling us that non-sexual stroking is calming and soothing and will get rid of stress and anxiety. For those of you with the time and the money I cannot recommend any treatment more highly than regular full body massages. If you live in or visit London check out NARI SADHURAM of HUMAN NATURE (13 Malvern Road, London, NW6 5PS, phone 020 7328 5452) who has been called "the best masseur in the world"

NARI SADHURAM

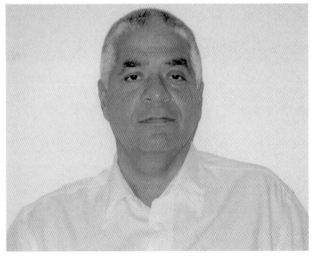

and is also known as "the man with the magic hands". NARI's clients include COURTNEY LOVE, JERRY HALL and LULU GUINNESS, the handbag queen and he will actually visit you in your own home which I think is the ultimate sensually pleasurable indulgence. NARI gives a wonderful toning and beautifying massage with essential oils which will leave your skin as soft as a baby's and frighten off any wobbly cellulite. He also specialises in Indian Head Massages which really clear your brain as well as stimulating hair growth. NARI says:

"What good is a massage?

Having given hundreds of massages over the years to all kinds of people, I can vouch for the fact that different people want different aspects of this therapy – from sports massage to simply enjoying being touched. But for me, a good massage has two essential qualities.

First of all it should make you not only feel better but it should bring tangible health benefits. There is no doubt that massage releases tight muscles and it helps to relieve back pain. And provided it is deep enough and properly targeted, massage boosts lymphatic system activity, thus preventing a build-up of cellulite in the thighs and upper arms. It also firms and tones the muscles and skin in a way that is quite different from the toning brought about by exercise. I'd go so far as to say that a good deep massage is essential during weight loss to tone and tighten up the skin.

Yet to say that massage is just good for your health is nonsense. There's a feel-good factor about massage that is equally important. Touch is one of the most important senses and the good feeling from the sensuality of massage can't be under-

estimated. I am not talking about sexuality here. There's obviously a big overlap between sex and massage simply because both involve one person stroking someone else's body. But the difference is crucial – and massage is about simply enjoying the feeling of being stroked and touched, of having attention focused on individual muscles and tendons, of being pummelled and stretched and cosseted all at once.

As to which is most important, I don't think you can separate these two aspects of a good massage. I always begin with dry brushing, for instance. I do it from the extremities, the hands and feet and shoulders, towards the heart because it pushes the lymph flow along and therefore has definite health benefits. But it also excites the capillaries just below the skin bringing the blood to the surface and is therefore extremely pleasurable.

I do a very deep massage on parts of the body – especially on the back where I actually jump up on the table astride the body for what's become known as the Steamroller. I also go as deep as possible on the upper thighs and upper arms. My motto is to use strokes that are just less than painful because these parts of the body are hard-worked and need deep strokes. Hitting this fine line brings maximum health benefits while the massage still remains pleasurable.

But it's not just these areas that get the attention. I massage almost every part of the body even the ears. I use various strokes such as light pummelling with the heels of the hand as well as combing or raking, using the fingers with feather touch massage on the thighs and the buttocks, even the back of the calves if the person is heavy. Like dry-brushing, feather touch strokes bring the blood to the surface, bringing a healthy glow as well as a pleasant sensation of well-being.

At the end, I'll always try to finish off with a head massage – something I brought from my childhood in India where I 'suffered' it at least once a week and was told that it would make my brains grow. I don't know about that – but it certainly promotes hair growth. And because the scalp is packed with nerve endings, a head massage, with its rubbing with palms and knuckles, the light brushing of the hair and scraping of the skin beneath, is intensely pleasurable.

So when you book a massage with me, don't expect one type of massage or another. Simply lay back and enjoy an experience that is good for your body, your mind and – I hope – your soul."

Now that you are exercising regularly (I hope!) you may need a "sports massage" from time to time to iron out any knots. If you have any stress in your life (unfortunately we all do sometimes even though you should try to avoid it

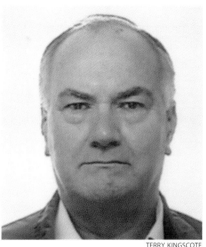

TERRY KINGSCOTE

as much as possible in order to become truly healthy) you will definitely be needing regular neuro-muscular massages to de stress you. The best practitioner I have found for this kind of strong, serious massage is TERRY KINGSCOTE, CSPhys (The Surgery, 7 Stanhope Mews West, South Kensington, SW7 5RB, phone 020 7835 0400/07714 643 403) who always succeeds in getting rid of all my exercise and stress related aches and pains in just one session. Here TERRY describes his techniques:

"Neuro-muscular massage

It is the best way to de-stress. It includes a combination of deep-tissue massage and a soothing but firm pressure which will calm the nerves and tone the muscles.

Sports massage

This breaks down painful knots and adhesions caused by stress and tension and stretches the muscles to give a feeling of better posture with more mobility and flexibility.

All types of Massage increase the blood flow and lymph circulation. This speeds up injury recovery, flushes out toxins and induces a feeling of relaxation and well-being."

Once you have learnt a little bit about massage technique you can pamper your partner regularly with a light home treatment with aromatherapy and essential oils from LUSH or THE BODY SHOP (stores nationwide). Keep it gentle: remember you are not NARI or TERRY and do keep your beautifully manicured and goddess like nails out of it!

Touch

23

TOUCHY FEELY

THERE is no more sensual pleasure than the feel of exquisite materials next to your skin: satin sheets, fluffy bath towels, fur (fake, please!) rugs in front of the fire. This is where silk and satin lingerie comes in: it just feels so much more sensually pleasurable than cotton or nylon against your naked skin.

The late great JANET REGER was the grande dame of British undies and visiting her Knightsbridge boutique (2 Beauchamp Place, London SW3 1NG, phone 020 7584 9360, www.janetreger.com) now run by her daughter ALIZA and manageress AVRIL SILVER is always a sensually pleasurable experience. You will especially enjoy rifling through JANET's latest "Naughty Janet" range! Wearing the right underpinnings will definitely make you feel like a goddess and your partner will thank you too.

Other manufacturers of sexy and strokeable skimpies include LA PERLA and LA SENZA, available in most big stores and ULTIMO (phone 0141 427 1010, www.ultimo.co.uk) make simply the best all-in-ones and padded bras if you need a little help in that area.

For those of you who need some inspiration on both what to wear and where to wear it, turn on THE LUXURY CHANNEL on satellite TV and check out what is truly sensually pleasurable in the big wide world.

By the way how does your actual skin feel to the touch? Does it feel as sensually pleasurable as your satin lingerie or reptilian? If you have followed my advice and are now having regular facials and beauty treatments, your face should now be feeling as soft as a baby's bottom. But what about *your* bottom and the rest of your body and limbs? You should use hand and body lotion twice a day, exfoliate at least once a week and use your DR DENESE Home Microdermabrasion Kit on any areas of your body that need it as well as on your face.

Your hands are particularly important as they are the one area of yourself that everybody can touch: I use CETUEM's Hand Exfoliant once a week, DR DENESE's Home Microdermabrasion Kit once a month and DR DENESE's Hand and Décolleté Serum daily to keep my hands (not to mention my décolleté) as soft and silky as a real goddess!

Touch

24

LOVE & ROMANCE
& A BIT OF SEX

IF you have taken all the advice of the preceding chapters you should be getting lots of loving by now (or at least plenty of offers!). Sex is good exercise and good for your health. However if you are unlucky enough to have a heart condition do be careful, take it easy and do not overdo the female pink Viagra!

Being in love makes you positively glow: "the look of love" is one of great beauty and people who are happily in love tend to be nicer to everyone around them. Now that you are as healthy, beautiful and goddess like as you deserve to be, you will probably have found a gorgeous lover. But how to keep him, that is the question? Keeping the romance in a relationship is not that easy: you have to always look, smell, taste, sound and feel your best. If you are married to or living with your man always change your clothes before he comes home if you have the chance; something soft and sensual is rather more attractive than your work out pants or gardening gear! Do not forget the Gold Spot just because you have been together for years (or you could try Choco Mints, chocolate flavoured breath strips containing no calories which are available from SALLY HAIR AND BEAUTY shops nationwide). Dabbing a bit of ESTÉE LAUDER's "Beyond Paradise" behind your ears takes two seconds and will bring out the goddess in you.

If you *are* married or "cohabiting" it is harder to look totally divine at all times, especially without make-up. This is where semi-permanent make-up comes in, as mentioned in Chapter 15. Men do not usually notice these subtle improvements, they just tend to say "she looks great without make-up" and that is exactly the effect we want to create.

Apart from looking after your personal hygiene and looks for your man, you will need to put him in the mood with romantic music, delicious wine or champagne and, of course, some aphrodisiac food. The best-known aphrodisiacs are shellfish, asparagus, wild mushrooms and truffles. Do not forget that the aphrodisiac effect takes half an hour or so to work so plan a leisurely meal when you are in the mood for love.

PETER STRINGFELLOW is a popular British celebrity and STRINGFELLOW'S CABARET OF ANGELS (16/19 Upper St Martin's Lane, WC2H 9EF, phone 020 7240 5534, www.stringfellows.com) is one of London's most erotic venues, full of girls who look like goddesses! The chefs at STRINGFELLOW'S (originally NICHOLAS BIBEVERIC and currently ROGER LEADBITTER) came up with the following four course aphrodisiac menu to tickle our fancies:

Suggested menu for love
- *Whitstable oysters served on ice with snails' eggs and Beluga caviar*
- *Asparagus garnished with fresh tomato and glazed with hollandaise sauce*
- *A combination of chicken, mussels and black truffles lightly steamed and presented on a warm vinaigrette*
- *A selection of tender vegetables sautéed in butter with new potatoes*
- *Pickled peaches soaked in honey with Royal Jelly*

You may like to play about with this menu and just use one or two of the aphrodisiac delicacies for each meal. Just remember to stay away from seriously unsexy foods like garlic (without the middle removed), raw onions, spinach, spare ribs and sweet corn if you want to impress your man, not put him off. You can eat those potentially embarrassing foods with the girls any time.

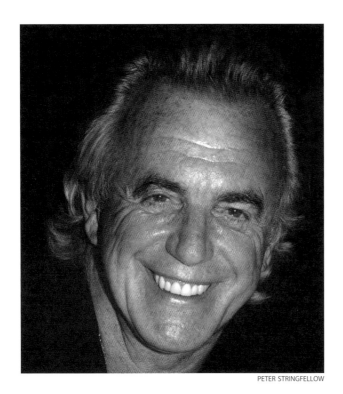

PETER STRINGFELLOW

Touch

25

GYNAECOLOGY
& SEX: THE SERIOUS STUFF

W E ladies need to look after ourselves inside and out and keep our female bits as healthy as the rest of us. All women of child-bearing age should have regular gynaecological check ups, smear tests and breast X-rays especially if there is a history of cancer in your family.

Harley Street gynaecologist MR MICHAEL BOWEN, FRCS, MRCOG, MRCP (The Hospital of St John's and St Elizabeth's, Grove End Road, NW8, phone 020 7467 8471) says:

GYNAECOLOGICAL AND OBSTETRIC ADVICE
from Mr Michael Bowen

Preventative health should start as early as possible. The basic messages about not smoking and healthy eating are probably the most important. Although it is not so apparent, smoking has a dramatic effect on a woman's gynaecological health, fertility and general health of her pregnancy.

Puberty
Healthy eating is a particularly important and difficult issue with adolescent women. At puberty, hormones change a girl's shape. She is particularly liable to lay down fat around the hips, thighs and buttocks. There is a tendency for the activity levels to change in some. With poor eating habits there is a risk of developing obesity, or at the other extreme, anorexia. Anorexia in particular can be especially dangerous, causing her periods to stop. If this state persists, the hormone levels will fall. Not

only is she at risk of the effects of hormone deficiency, but also premature ovarian failure and subsequent early menopause. If it is possible to correct this with a healthy diet, the menstrual cycle will return but often some time later.

Puberty is associated with a rise in hormones. Apart from enhancing secondary sexual characteristics, they also can bring some unwelcome effects such as premenstrual tension, period pains and teenage spots.

If these are especially troublesome, you should consult your doctor who will be able to advise you about the full range of treatments now available. Some success has been reported in treating PMT with vitamin B12 or evening primrose oil. The combined oral contraceptive pill has been used to good effect in treating a number of teenagers with hormone-related prob-

lems. It works by abolishing their natural hormone cycle and the fluctuations in hormone levels, and in addition provides contraception. The combined oral contraceptive pill has revolutionised the lives of women, allowing women some choice about when they start a family.

There have been some questions about how safe it is and whether it can make one more prone to illnesses such as blood clots and breast cancer. It is said that the pill is not dangerous but some women are dangerous when taking the pill. A good example of this is the risks associated with a healthy woman with no significant family history taking the pill at the age of 25 compared with a women who has a family history of thrombosis or factor V Leiden deficiency who is obese and smokes heavily. Obviously, in the latter group the pill has some significant risks associated with it and if one falls into this category then often a doctor will advise about using an alternative method of contraception.

The combined oral contraceptive pill is effective in stopping ovulation and preventing pregnancy, however it provides little in the way of barrier protection from sexually transmitted infections and it is advisable if you are not in a stable relationship to continue to use a barrier method of contraception. This will not only prevent the transmission of sexually transmitted infections that can harm your fertility but also infections that may harm your cervix and cause cervical disease in the future.

It is important to note that not everyone can take the pill effectively and sometimes some couples will experience an accident with their contraception. The obvious result of unprotected intercourse is the risk of pregnancy. For such situations there is emergency contraception or commonly termed "morning after pill". The term "morning after pill" is particularly bad and misleading because emergency contraception in tablet form is available up to 48 and 72 hours after unprotected sex and it is possible to provide emergency contraception up to five days after any episode by using an intrauterine contraceptive device.

Lately, emergency contraception in the form of a pill has been available over the counter at pharmacies. This causes a withdrawal bleed and some discomfort and is successful in preventing pregnancies in most cases.

Pregnancy

It is said that women spend half of their time worrying about if they could have an unplanned pregnancy and the rest of the time worrying about if they will have a pregnancy when they wish to have one.

If you are trying to become pregnant, I would suggest forgetting the idea of trying to have sex at the right time; although it is advantageous and important to have regular unprotected sex in order to conceive, it is by no means essential. There is little evidence to suggest that forcing yourself to have intercourse according to your cycle is likely to significantly improve your chances of conception. We are essentially programmed to be more interested in sex when we are at our most fertile but suddenly watching the clock to decide when you have intercourse runs the risk of turning what should be a pleasurable activity into a stressful ordeal. Generally, it is important to have a healthy diet, take regular exercise and take folic acid supplements. It is important to take these in the first six weeks of pregnancy and for most women they will not necessarily know they are pregnant for the first three weeks of pregnancy. As a rule, 90% of couples will achieve conception within the first 12 months and if you have not conceived after a period of having regular intercourse in this time, then it is worth having some investigations.

Understandably, older women sometimes feel the pressure to have such investigations done much sooner as after the age of 35, natural fertility begins to decline and the risk of Down's syndrome and chromosomal abnormalities increase at a faster rate. As a woman ages, having babies later in life means that medical disorders such as high blood pressure and diabetes become more common. There is a risk once these have been diagnosed when this is combined with pregnancy. However, the good news is that for mature mothers who are fit and healthy and do not smoke, their risks are not that much different from 20-year-olds. Women having babies at an older age should be reassured that once they have established they can get pregnant and that the pregnancy is healthy, their performance in pregnancy and labour should have little difference from women considerably younger.

Becoming pregnant is a complex process which involves sperm getting to the right place at the right time and an egg being in the right place at the right time to meet the sperm. When analysing every single step of the way, not only does it become a complex and carefully co-ordinated event, but also it is a wonder that anybody actually achieves it as frequently as they do!

The investigations principally involve investigating every part of the journey, as all the blocks need to be in place in order to achieve a conception. Subfertility affects one in seven couples and of these, approximately a third of the time it is due to male factors, a third of the time due to female factors and a third of the time it is a combination of the two.

After examining every single stage of the conception process your gynaecologist will be able to advise you on how to improve your chances of becoming pregnant. Ultimately, in vitro fertilisation or IVF is a process which bypasses the fallopian tubes. The sperm and egg are mixed outside the womb – in vitro – i.e. in glass. This is then replaced in the womb once the egg is fertilised and becomes an embryo. This is an area which is rapidly advancing and attracts some degree of controversy pushing back the moral and ethical boundaries.

Once you become pregnant one of the commonest complaints is of morning sickness. This is extremely common and quite normal but occasionally if vomiting is excessive it is worth visiting your doctor who will ensure that you do not have a urinary tract infection and probably refer you for an ultrasound scan to confirm that you have a healthy intrauterine pregnancy, as vomiting is more common with twin pregnancies and a particular type of condition in the placenta. There is some recent evidence to suggest that morning sickness may be a healthy sign in pregnancy. This can be extremely troublesome and can cause some degree of misery for women but fortunately it only usually lasts for the first 14 weeks. Various remedies have been tried for morning sickness such as anti-sickness tablets and dry ginger which have varying degrees of success in women.

One controversial area in the first 14 weeks of pregnancy is how much alcohol you are allowed to drink. There is no doubt that drinking large amounts of alcohol is detrimental to your baby and in extreme circumstances can lead to foetal alcohol syndrome. Advice throughout the world varies as to how much is safe to drink and, to be honest, there are very few large-scale studies which give any real indication as to whether one glass of wine a day is likely to be harmful to your baby. It is worth checking with your doctor what the current recommendation is although it is always rather surprising given the number of babies that are conceived under the influence of alcohol!

During pregnancy it is important to ensure you are healthy and regular check-ups with the doctor or midwife have a useful role. Not only is it an opportunity for you to be seen and ensure that you *are* healthy and are not showing signs of any underlying disease but it is also an opportunity for you to ask questions and be given reassurance about changes you may see in your body. Recently, more and more women ask whether they should invest in having the baby privately or stay within the NHS. This is something which is worth discussing with your doctor but private care for obstetrics is exceptionally expensive and is difficult to find outside London. During the pregnancy it is important to arm yourself with information, particularly if you have had any complications in the past or a family history of any disorders. Very often there are no hard and fast rules about what to do in pregnancy, merely a chance of experiencing particular events if you choose one option or another. It is important to discuss these with the doctors and midwives who may be involved in your care.

Labour and Delivery

Unfortunately, in pregnancy one does always have to be prepared for the unexpected as situations can change very quickly. Elective Caesarean section births are on the increase. This is where the mother decides to have her baby by Caesarean section rather than have a vaginal delivery. In some cases this is the safest way to have the baby and in others this is an option with advantages and disadvantages.

On the whole Caesarean section involves a seven inch cut in the bikini line and can take longer to recover from compared to a straightforward normal delivery. However, for some women it is preferable to have a Caesarean rather than a difficult and complicated forceps or assisted delivery.

One such dilemma is when a woman has had a Caesarean section in which case her chances of having a vaginal delivery the next time are approximately 60%. This may be a quick, straightforward vaginal delivery with little in the way of trauma, in which case the woman will recover very quickly. On the other hand there is a 40% chance she will require an emergency Caesarean section during labour which has a greater risk than having a planned Caesarean section. During labour there is a risk the scar from the previous Caesarean section can separate. Occasionally this may be an emergency situation.

This poses a very difficult issue for many couples as the choice following a Caesarean section delivery is (1) to have a planned Caesarean section which gives some degree of certainty but does not have the advantages of having a straightforward vaginal delivery; however it does not have the disadvantages of (2) having an emergency Caesarean section or of a complicated vaginal delivery. Unfortunately, nature and your body do not necessarily read your birth plan and it is very important to keep an open mind and share your thoughts and anxieties with the people around you.

Sex

During a vaginal delivery it is sometimes necessary to perform an episiotomy and some woman will experience vaginal and perineal tears. A common sequelae to this is having pain after childbirth during intercourse. This can be extremely distressing for a couple. Added to tiredness, exhaustion

and a reduction in hormones during breast-feeding it is not surprising that many woman lose all interest in sex.

It is important to discuss these issues with your partner. If you experience vaginal dryness and soreness in the vagina which can sometimes be associated with breast-feeding it is worth approaching your GP who will be able to prescribe you some cream or lubricant jelly that will ease the situation.

There is a word of caution here: if one does use oils as a lubricant you have to be mindful that they can impair the integrity of latex condoms and reduce their effectiveness. Breast-feeding itself is not a reliable method of contraception and if you are not planning on having another baby immediately it is worth thinking about an appropriate method of birth control.

The biggest sex organ we possess is the brain and it is in this area where most problems with sex occur. Men too can be traumatised by childbirth and this can manifest itself in a number of ways.

If your partner appears to have lost interest in you for any reason, after giving birth or whatever, use your feminine wiles and manipulation to get him back on track: it is essential to get out the Janet Reger or La Perla underwear and scented candles. You should devise a "sex menu" which pleases you both.

Adopting Kama Sutra positions will not necessarily give you a fulfilling sex life. Close your eyes and focus and concentrate on the sensual experience. Foreplay is all important, particularly if penetrative sex has been painful but you want to return to it. Psychologically women often do not want to be pro active in sex so they have to find some way to communicate their needs to their other half. It is so important to communicate: people should talk more.

SEXUALLY TRANSMITTED DISEASES

from Dr Anna, Lady Brocklebank

Safe sex is all important in today's world, whatever your age. Here is a report from DR ANNA, LADY BROCKLEBANK, BM (St George's Hospital, London, SW17).

"Very nice people catch syphilis – Debretts is full of them – Bonaparte, Beethoven – all great syphilis sufferers." So said one teacher in our one and only lecture on STDs during medical school. The point being that STDs have no class boundaries – they are entirely democratic.

The fact that as students we only had one lecture on the matter demonstrates how low on the list of medical priorities STDs were and, sadly, still are for some people. Even today you will find the STD clinic tucked discreetly away from the more glamorous departments of any hospital.

So long as people are having sex, there will be sexual infections even though most of them can be prevented and treated very easily – so easily that my old boss told me that by 1950 when Penicillin was easily available, consultant specialists of STDs thought that they would be out of a job and finally syphilis and gonorrhoea would be eradicated. They needn't have worried about unemployment – far from being eliminated, the incidence of STDs continued to climb in a way unheard of before. ⁰It seemed that knowing there was a treatment for hitherto untreatable illnesses coupled with the 60s philosophy of free love led to an apparent disregard for the risks of contracting a nasty little disease.

In spite of sexual education and the apparent sophistication of today's youth, there is still a huge amount of misunderstanding around the subject of STDs, and the incidence of these infections continues to soar; for no other reason than laziness and ignorance. Most women have no problems having regular cervical smears in order to prevent cancer so you would have thought that they would find it just as easy to have a quick swab check with every change of partner. I suspect the reason why people have difficulties acknowledging the needs for STDs check ups is nothing more than good old prejudice. We in GU Medicine are still very much the poor relation in most hospitals with even our colleagues looking down their noses in our direction. One cardiologist whom I dated a few years ago even went as far as to suggest I was not a proper doctor and, therefore, might feel at sea accompanying him to a medical dinner.

And yet having an untreated STD cannot only wreck your health, current and long term, but it can destroy relationships. An STD is not the ideal love gift.

What are the common STDs seen today?

Chlamydia, gonorrhoea, herpes, genital warts, syphilis and HIV.

Where do they come from?

Genital infections have been described even since records started to be kept although in the distant past individual infections were often thought of as one disease. Syphilis, which stands apart in terms of its symptoms, has many stories accounting for its appearance. The commonest theory is that Christopher Columbus and his colleagues picked up the infection from the inhabitants of the New World and brought it back to Europe.

Mythology has it that Aphrodite, the Greek Goddess of love, fell in love with a shepherd boy called Syphilis. However when he rejected her amorous advances – preferring instead his shepherdess girlfriend – Aphrodite, consumed with rage, struck him down with a horrific disease which eventually ravaged his whole body – this disease was thereafter named after the shepherd – Syphilis.

What do STDs do to the body?

Chlamydia Is a little intracellular organism which frequently causes no symptoms at all. This makes it a particularly nasty little infection as it will often go untreated. If left untreated in a woman it can cause infertility and in a man inflammation of the testicles and/or prostate gland. In the last ten years the incidence of chlamydia has risen from 3% of all boys between 17 and 25 to 20%. That is one in five boys! Use of condoms considerably decreases the chance of contracting the disease but since it so often doesn't cause any symptoms, sexually active people should have tests with every change of sexual partner… and use condoms – prevention is better than cure.

Pregnant women can pass chlamydia on to their baby causing eye problems and/or pneumonia so a chlamydia test is advisable with pregnancy. Fortunately chlamydia is easily treated with antibiotics.

Gonorrhoea This particular infection is not currently quite so common as chlamydia, possibly because it frequently causes symptoms in men which encourage them to get it dealt with. "Pissing razor blades" is how men often describe the symptoms and a nasty yellow discharge pours from the penis. Occasionally men will insist that they only have a "cold" in their willy and not an STD. I answer that when it sneezes it's a cold and until then we'll call it gonorrhoea. Like chlamydia, gonorrhoea if left untreated can cause infertility in women in addition to many other problems including arthritis. Men are frequently reluctant to go to a "special" clinic, so ladies, if you notice your man has a "cold in his penis" or anything else that looks odd – *bring him down* to the clinic with you.

Herpes The herpes virus is responsible for not only genital herpes but also "cold sores" commonly found around the mouth. Most sufferers of cold sores are not unduly concerned with the matter and certainly don't consider themselves as having a sexual disease. However, should they indulge in the popular pastime of oral sex, they can pass the herpes virus onto their partners' genitals thereby giving them genital herpes which frequently causes emotional distress and anxiety.

Frankly, if I were to have herpes I would much rather have it somewhere hidden like below my belt rather than all over my face – but such is the western attitude to "matters down below" that the vast majority of herpes sufferers seem to view genital herpes as something infinitely more horrifying. The recurrent nature of herpes is often the cause of much distress although with appropriate long-term treatment this need not be a problem. As with all infections, condoms help prevent contracting or spreading the virus. But remember, condoms give safer sex not 100% safe sex.

Herpes in pregnancy must be treated and it is often advised that a caesarean section should be performed in the case of a woman having an outbreak at the time of delivery. Herpes in pregnancy should not be a problem as long as the GP and the antenatal staff are all aware of the situation. It is vital that the information is present on all notes particularly the antenatal notes.

Genital warts These are caused by the Human Papiloma Virus and are nearly always the result of sexual contact. They often go unnoticed in women as the female anatomy is such that a woman has to be a bit of a contortionist with a mirror to have a good look. I am, however, surprised by how many women (usually quite young) get their boyfriends to double up as a gynaecologist.

There are over 80 different types of genital warts and the major concern regarding women is that two of the types (16 and 18) are associated with pre malignant disease of the cervix. This is not a problem as long as the woman remembers her regular cervical smear check up.

During pregnancy, warts usually run riot and the normal treatment of Warticon cream is not recommended. Most patients are advised to do nothing until after the delivery when the warts will usually diminish in number and it is also safe to treat.

Syphilis My old boss used to say, "If you understand syphilis, you understand all of medicine". What he meant was that untreated syphilis can affect every system in the human body. The initial symptoms are a non painful genital ulcer followed six weeks later by a flu like illness and rash. These symptoms are quite easy to miss. Years later if untreated, syphilis may cause profound nervous, mental and physical disturbances which are not frequently seen these days as syphilis is so easy to treat. However, the disease must first be identified – so get along to your STD clinic and have a blood test.

The pregnant woman can pass syphilis to her unborn child resulting in a very serious illness for the baby. In most western countries this is avoided by every woman being tested at her first antenatal appointment. However mistakes are still made. I am thinking of the wife of a Professor of Medicine (now retired). Because she was the wife of a medically "important" man, she did not have the usual blood tests in the antenatal clinic. They obviously thought she was too "nice" a person to "have anything like that". Well of course it was most embarrassing for all concerned that at 32 weeks pregnant, she was identified as having syphilis. I saw her in clinic where she was treated and fortunately gave birth to a healthy child.

HIV AIDS This is one condition that most people are familiar with as there has been heavy media involvement. It is no longer associated just with homosexuality – like all

the other STDs it has no social boundaries and is not class conscious. Horrifyingly there are still people who are HIV positive having sex without condoms but more startling still are the "virus chasers" who actively seek out HIV positive partners so that they too can contract the disease. (The mental gymnastics required to understand that state of mind is too much for most of us.) However, having contracted the virus, the news is good and getting better. With the drugs available there is no reason why most HIV positive people can't live an active life with a normal life span. But prevention is still better than cure. So **USE CONDOMS.**

Do you have to have sexual intercourse in order to pick up an STD?

This depends on whether or not you embrace President Clinton's definition of sexual intercourse.

Years ago a friend of mine employed a professional lady to play "under the table" games at his stag night – the most popular game being "how long can you keep a straight face while receiving fellatio?" Like Clinton, none of them felt they had had proper sexual intercourse and were therefore very surprised to find out they had all contracted gonorrhoea from an infection in the girl's mouth. The same can happen with herpes, chlamydia and syphilis.

So the message I would like to give is to go out and have sex – it's fun and it keeps you young, but please be safe – a condom can literally save your life.

SEX ADDICTION

from Dr Anna, Lady Brocklebank

It is just as important to be sexually healthy mentally as physically. If you suffer from sex addiction, as MICHAEL DOUGLAS allegedly once did before meeting his Welsh goddess CATHERINE ZETA-JONES, or have any serious sexual hang-ups, you will probably need professional help. Here is DR BROCKLEBANK again:

When Michael Douglas announced to the world that he was a sex addict, I thought, "yeah, right – just the latest fad out of America to excuse men who can't keep their pants on". A view strengthened by Bill Clinton and Robbie Williams also being given the same diagnosis – surely they're just a lot of randy boys with no self control?

And then I was asked to see a German patient. A physically attractive man in his early thirties. He owned a company employing over 200 people – mostly women – all of whom he had had sex with – to the detriment of working conditions. Very Clintonesque, I thought. Then he told me that he was quite incapable of going through the day without a "quickie". Even if he was driving on the motorway – he would have to stop the car and proposition a girl at a petrol station. This is where the story gets nasty; if he couldn't find a girl who was willing to have sex, he would feel a compulsion to rape one. He told me he just couldn't stop himself after which he would feel incredibly guilty and full of remorse. The guilt would make him feel so bad that it was like an "empty hole which he had to fill" – he then needed to anaesthetise himself and his emotions. And guess what anaesthetised his emotions and blotted out the bad feelings best of all? More sex. The sex, he said, gave him a big high but it was never very long before the guilt and remorse set in again. This behaviour of his meant that work relations within his company were fraught with difficulties, and although he yearned for a stable relation-

ship with his children, he was seemingly incapable of conducting a monogamous relationship for more than a few weeks. He had put his physical being at risk by having unprotected sex with an enormous amount of casual girlfriends. By luck more than good judgement he was HIV negative but nevertheless had had syphilis, herpes, gonorrhoea and chlamydia and the only reason he was not in jail for rape was that so far, none of his victims had prosecuted him. He cried with his head in his hands and pleaded for someone or something to stop his compulsive behaviour. It was at that point for me, the penny dropped.

I recognised and was only too aware of the cycle of addiction that he described so vividly and the misery that accompanied that cycle. The need to anaesthetise oneself with drink or drugs or as in this case, sex. The instant high – the fix – followed by guilt followed by a further compulsion to anaesthetise oneself again. A cycle that can only go in one direction, down – in spite of the fact that at times you can fool yourself and others that you have things under control. This is the point with addictions, the addict can't control them.

So what made my patient a sex addict as opposed to a jolly Casanova? Well, the jolly Casanova does not have his life ruined by his pre-occupation with sex. He is still able to perform his professional duties, he is able to maintain social and personal relationships, and he is not vulnerable to prosecution by the law. The addict on the other hand, is driven by his addiction – it comes before work relationships, the law of the land and family. Addiction is without doubt the most generally destructive disease. Affecting not only the victim but those around him.

Having been convinced that the concept of sex addiction did exist as opposed to the general promiscuous nature of the male species, I then looked at the nature of certain sexual behavioural patterns to see if the addiction cycle applied to them. In par-

ticular I considered the paraphilias – Greek for "beyond the norm" – behavioural patterns that many consider to be deviant. The paraphilias include:

- **Sadism** – pleasure from mistreating others
- **Masochism** – pleasure from being mistreated
- **Fetishism** – sexual pleasure from non-living objects e.g. shoes
- **Frotteurism** – pleasure from rubbing against a non consenting women – commonly done in crowded tube carriages
- **Transvestism** – sexual pleasure from wearing women's clothes

The list is endless and limited only by man's imagination or lack of it.

Considering the subject of paraphilias initially led me to collapse in school girl giggles and be aghast in equal measures. The conservative MP who had been found dead, hanging from the ceiling with an orange in his mouth and wearing a French maid's uniform, exhibiting transvestism and masochism, staggered the nation and did nothing to repair the Tories' reputation for sleaze. More recently the governmental advisor to Iraq whose dominatrix mistress revealed that his idea of fun was a rubber wet suit and gas mask – pictures provided for the tabloids.

After the initial disbelief and hilarity the question remained why should these usually successful men want to humiliate themselves and expose themselves to public ridicule, causing collapse of their professional and personal life and in some cases death?

Over the years I have interviewed a number of these people. There is a sense of distress within these individuals. In other words, they typically recognise the symptoms as negatively impacting their lives but feel as if they are unable to control them. As a rule they do not go to the doctor's office complaining of their sexual practice – usually they will not particularly wish to stop doing something they enjoy. It is often their partner who feels she can't handle the practice or wants to know more about why her partner wishes to behave in a particular fashion. In some instances the female partner is willing to play along and in some cases will actively enjoy the activity. This is particularly the case in the surprisingly common practice of sado masochism. Ten years ago I met a girl from a well known aristocratic family at Langhams restaurant. She was wearing white PVC boots with matching mini skirt and told me her working name was Countess Zena. She had a timeshare in a dungeon in Marble Arch where she would give her clients a thoroughly hard time for £500 and for £1,000 they wouldn't sit down for a week. She added that she was very busy and very rich with a very strong right arm from wielding the whip. It is of note that in nearly all cases, the person with the paraphilias is male. Many papers written on the subject confirm my view that the exception to this is sado masochism. It is also remarkable that of the men exhibiting deviant behaviour, most are from the upper echelons of society and successful. Politicians and lawyers seem particularly partial to unconventional practices although this may be an impression gained through the tabloid press who may seek to expose this particular class of person on a fairly regular basis.

Whatever the sexual practice, on the whole the behavioural pattern is laid down in the early years of development, many experts saying that sexual patterns are established by the age of eight. I found this to be well illustrated by a successful politician who told me that at the age of seven he was playing on a rope swing and somersaulted several times so that his limbs became tangled up in the ropes. To his amazement and bewilderment, he had an erotic experience which he has spent the rest of his life recreating. Preferring

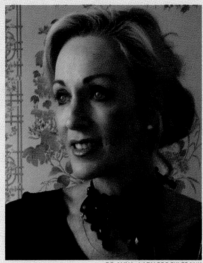

DR ANNA, LADY BROCKLEBANK

something more sophisticated than a rope swing he now has a leather and metal chastity belt which he likes to wear before asking his partner to truss him up like a Xmas turkey.

For those of you who have read Tom Sharpe's *Blott on the Landscape* or seen the TV series made of it starring George Cole as the politician who enjoyed being tied up while wearing a baby's nappy and bonnet, you will appreciate how ridiculous the vision of this behaviour is. But just consider what an overwhelming compulsion the person must feel that he should compromise himself in such a way (it is interesting to note that a recurring feature of many paraphilias is humiliation and degradation).

These sexual practices while not in themselves harmful or illegal are frequently responsible for the break up of relationships, families and destruction of careers. Listening to patients describing the "high" that they feel followed by remorse and humiliation after indulging in their activity sounds remarkably like other addictive processes.

Some paraphilias are obviously less harmful than others. A love of being tied up and spanked is not in the same league as exhibitionism (exposing genitalia to a female) or voyeurism (peeping tom). The latter two being illegal and by definition involving non consenting individuals. But like all addictions, these activities are dynamic and what can start as a bit of fun with a hair brush can develop into full blown criminal activity – just as the marijuana smoker may turn into a heroin addict. And the activity can still be criminal even if all parties consent. The case of R v Brown involved five consenting adult males who nailed each other's testicles to a piece of wood. They were each found guilty of GBH. Although contentious, this case has not yet been overruled.

So, you might say, what is wrong with a bit of imaginative hanky panky? The answer is nothing so long as it doesn't interfere with relationships, work or family in a negative fashion. If it does, then like all addictions it must be treated. Personally I loathe the 12 step program involved in Alcoholics Anonymous and Narcotics Anonymous but it does work for most people. There are now groups for Sex and Love Addicts Anonymous which apparently have great success – although the idea of a room full of sex addicts all talking to each other about sex seems to be a bit self-defeating. Other therapies include cognitive behavioural therapy (CBT), hypnotherapy, psychotherapy, acupuncture and a selection of rehabilitation units. Michael Douglas is now evidently happily married to the lovely Catherine Zeta-Jones – with his sex addiction no longer a problem – whether it was 12 steps that helped him or just finding a soul mate is sadly something most of us will never know.

Touch

26

SEX
THE FUN STUFF

ARE you "lover ready", as CARRIE so subtly puts it in *Sex and the City*? If you are going to get naked with some gorgeous hunk (your lawn boy or whomever!) you must be looking your absolute best. Have you got rid of any pimples, had your roots done, attended to your armpits and had your bikini, Brazilian or Bollywood wax? Have you had your semi permanent make-up applied by or DAWN CRAGG, including your nipples coloured? In that case go for it.

Exercises and techniques

Making love is great exercise as well as our favourite sensual pleasure. This does not necessarily mean you have to swing from the chandeliers or indulge in marathon sex sessions all the time. If you want to improve your technique and build up your stamina try American favourite, "SEXERCISES", included in VALERIE AUSTIN's online book *Hypnosex*:

SEXERCISES
from Valerie Austin

Exercise for both women and men is very important to a good sexual relationship. Vaginal exercises for the woman entail simply squeezing your vaginal muscles together. Scrotum exercises for the man are well worth the effort. For both sexes the exercises take less than a minute but it can make all the difference to responses in love-making. Other exercises meanwhile help to firm up important areas.

Scrotum Exercise
There are several factors that help a man to attain an erection. It is important to have good blood circulation. This can be improved by regular exercise, especially exercising the muscle between your legs behind the scrotum. This is where the blood flow is compressed, helping to engorge the penis.

The man can regularly exercise this muscle by pretending to hold back his water. When he goes to the toilet he can stop the flow by using the muscle. The man needs to exercise this muscle about 25 times a day, every day, and within a very short space of time the strengthening of it will help him in love-making.

Vaginal Exercise
This is very similar to the scrotum exercise. You tense the bunch of muscles in the way you would if you were trying to stop yourself from urinating and hold them for five seconds and then let go, 15 times a day. This exercise will firm the muscles up instead of them sagging with age and you will find you have more control in the sexual regions. This is a very good exercise to begin if you are over 40.

Here is another physical exercise that will tone up those sexual muscles.
For women Stand erect with your feet apart. Squat about halfway down, hands behind your neck. Thrust your sex organ area downward and backward as far as it will go and hold for six seconds.

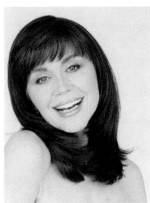

DR AVA CADELL

Perhaps you are already super fit, "lover ready", willing and able but want to improve your love life, enhance your relationships and enjoy greater sexual fulfilment? In that case do read our hypnotherapist VALERIE AUSTIN's fascinating online book, *Hypnosex* at: www.hypnosexinthecity.com

Now it is over to the world renowned DR AVA CADELL, HOLLYWOOD's "Master Sexpert" for some little lovemaking tips:

"Here are some tips for you as you go off on your sensual sexual exploration. Get yourself in the mood by stimulating all five of your senses – here are a few suggestions:

- *For your sense of taste: make sure you have all your favourite finger foods and beverages available nearby, such as strawberries, grapes and chocolates… A true aphrodisiac. Feed each other before lovemaking as part of your foreplay.*
- *Sound: play sexy music, use erotic talk and don't forget to scream, "Yes, Yes, Yes" whenever your lover gets it right.*
- *Sight: Make love in front of a mirror, decorate with flowers, dress up in sexy lingerie.*
- *Smell: Wear your lover's favourite fragrance, light some incense or scented candles.*
- *Touch: caress your lover with fabrics like feathers, silk, velvet, satin, latex, leather or even metal chains.*
- *The final tip – tell your lover to take up juggling because he's going to need to work on his co-ordination to master sexual techniques but it's well worth the effort and mighty fun learning!*

Don't forget what MAE WEST said: 'too much of a good thing is wonderful!'"

So there you have it. Lovemaking is one of the few times when you can indulge in chocolate chomping without feeling guilty: after all, it is not for you but for your loverrr, is it not? If you do decide to take DR AVA's advice and feed him chocolate, the most sensually pleasurable choccies I have found in the whole of the capital are by PIERRE MARCOLINI (6 Lancer Square, Kensington, W8 4EH, phone 020 7795 6611, www.pierremarcolini.co.uk)

By the way if you really, really want to know everything there is to know about sex and more, visit DR AVA's sites at www.avacadell.com or www.sexpert.com. You can then learn how to master advanced sexual techniques and become a true sex goddess. You can even read all about DR AVA's latest discovery, "the Trigasm, a oneness with the universe". "There hasn't been an innovation like it since the discovery of the G-Spot by DR ERNEST GRAFENBERG in the 50s!" breathes sultry DR AVA.

We are always being promised "enhanced sexual pleasure" these days with tabloid glamour girls like SALLY-ANNE JONES and DENISE HEWITT having G-Spot and "vaginal rejuvenation" operations respectively. Good for you if you want to improve your sex life but do consult your doctor first and go to a respected surgeon.

Finally never forget that sex should be fun, as well as romantic, passionate and sensually pleasurable. After all the Great British Press are fond of dubbing sexy people "fun loving". How about a trip to JANET REGER or AGENT PROVOCATEUR (16 Pont Street, Belgravia, SW1X 9EN, phone 020 7235 0229) to buy some fun garments to spice up your sex life? You will never truly appreciate the joys of fully-fashioned black seamed stockings and lacy suspenders until you try them. But do find out discreetly what your man likes before going the whole hog with the French maid's outfit or nurse's uniform! Some men do not even like nightdresses and negligees and prefer their ladies to wear giant tee shirts to bed: "à chacun son goût".

EPILOGUE

I HOPE you have enjoyed reading this book and are now a fully fledged Health Goddess. You will need to maintain the good results you have achieved, living a stress free, healthy and beautiful life. Now you have found them, enjoy your Sensual Pleasures FOREVER.

LIST OF CONTRIBUTORS

ACCUVISION, 42–48 New King's Road, London, SW6 4LS, 020 7736 2020

AUSTIN, VALERIE, 118 Piccadilly, London W1, 020 7702 4900, www.valerieaustin.com

BERBATOVCI, CARLO, The Café Delancey

BIBEVERIC, NICHOLAS, Chef, Stringfellow's, 16–19 Upper St Martin's Lane, WC2H 9EF, 020 7240 5534, www.stringfellows.com

BIRD, HEATHER, HB Health, 48 Harley St, London W1G 7JQ, 020 7323 1388 and 12 Beauchamp Place, Knightsbridge, SW3 1NZ, 020 7838 0765

BLACK, SHARON, 07767 296 690

BORISSOV, VALENTIN, 118 Piccadilly, London, W1, 020 7569 6815

BOWEN, MICHAEL, FRCS, MRCOG, MRCP, The Hospital of St John's and St Elizabeth's, Grove End Road, London, NW8, 020 7467 8471

BOWLER, PATRICK, Dr, MS.BS, LRCP, MRCS, DRCOG The Court House Clinic, 30B Wimpole Street, London, W1, 0870 850 3456

BROCKLEBANK, ANNA, LADY, Dr, BM, St George's Hospital, London, SW17

BROSI, HENRY, Executive Chef, The Dorchester, 53 Park Lane, London W1A 2HJ, 020 7629 8888

BRUNI, GEORGINA, Hot Gossip's Editor in Chief, www.hotgossip.co.uk

CADELL, AVA, Dr, www.avacadell.com

CHAPMAN, JACQUELINE, RGN ONC, 020 8300 7616, www.bellydancer.org.uk

CLARKE, NICKY, 130 Mount Street, London, W1K 3NY, 020 7491 4700

COEN, CARINA, Mercarina Private Clinic, 56 Seymour Street, London W1H 7JJ, 020 7724 0514, www.mercarina.com

COLOUR ME BEAUTIFUL, 66 The Business Centre, 15–17 Ingate Place, London SW8 3NS, 020 7627 5211, www.cmb.co.uk

COSTELLO, ANN, The Dorchester, 53 Park Lane, London W1A 2HJ, 020 7629 8888

COX, PETER, Nutritionist, HB Health, 48 Harley St, London W1G 7JQ, 020 7323 1388 and 12 Beauchamp Place, Knightsbridge, SW3 1NZ, 020 7838 0765

DALE-ELIASHIV, ORNA, 07747 185 318, orna59@yahoo.com

DE CARLE, JOHN, Opticians and contact lens practitioners, 15 Brook's Mews, Mayfair, W1K 4DS, 020 7408 1208

D'ARCY, DEBORAH, 07939 479 420

DRYSDALE, WILLIAM, Hot Gossip's Canadian fitness correspondent, www.hotgossip.co.uk

ECOLE DE SKI INTERNATIONALE, Val Thorens, Les Trois Vallees, France – Brise, Head Teacher

EVANS, JOANNE, The Medical Rooms, The Soma Centre, 2–24 High Street Kensington, W8 4TP, 020 7361 0616, 07710 381 438

FERRALL-PEEVEY, LAURA, Air Brush Tanning, 07867 610 045 www.bronzetallulah.co.uk

FIONA, Accuvision, 42–48, New King's Road, London, SW6 4LS, 020 7736 2020

FREIBERGER, MALCOLM, BDS, LDSRCS, MFGDP, 9a Portland Place, London, W1B 1PR, 020 7636 8495

GINNINGS, JANET, Janet Ginnings Salon, 45 Curzon Street, Mayfair, W1, 020 7499 2767, www.janetginnings.co.uk

GLANCEY, LUCY, Dr, MRCS, Grove Clinic, Grove Farm, Grove Hill, Langham, Essex, CO4 5PJ, 0870 458 5483, www.glanceymedical.co.uk

GULAMALI, SHIRAZ, Dr, BDS, LDSRCS, MSC, FDSRCPS, 12 Upper Wimpole Street, London, W1G 6LW, 020 7486 2466, 020 7935 9511, www.gumsandimplants.co.uk

THE HALE CLINIC 7 Park Crescent, London, W1B 1PF, 020 7631 0156, www.haleclinic.com

HART, RICHARD, Dr, GP 020 8952 5536, 07956 384 667

HENDERSON, VERONIQUE, Colour Me Beautiful, 66 The Business Centre, 15–17 Ingate Place, London SW8 3NS, 020 7627 5211, www.cmb.co.uk

HILL, AL, 07973 213 091, al.hill@btinternet.com

HOLMES PLACE, 020 7786 7300, www.holmesplace.com

HOLMES PLACE, FULHAM, Normand Park, Lillie Road, SW6 7ST, 020 7471 0450 – David Thomas, Alun Thomas

HOOLEY, JOAN, Anita Arun Representation, 020 7379 6840

HOPLEY, JILL, The Hale Clinic, 7 Park Crescent, London, W1B 1PF, 020 7631 0156, www.haleclinic.com

ION, LUCIAN, FRCS (Plast), 129 Harley Street, London, W1G 6BA, 020 7224 5434, www.aesthetic-plastic-surgery.co.uk

JACKSON, CINDY, www.cindyjackson.com

KARIDIS, ALEX, MD, FRCS, The Hospital of St John and St Elizabeth, 60 Grove End Road, London, NW8 9NK, 020 7432 8727, www.nipntuck.co.uk

KILLICK, PAUL, Dancesport Studio, 57 Pont Street, London, SW1X 0BD, 020 7589 3071, www.paulkillick.com

KINGSCOTE, TERRY, CS Phys, The Surgery, 7 Stanhope Mews West, South Kensington, SW7 5RB, 020 7835 0400, 07714 643 403

LATIMER-SAYER, EDWARD, BSc, MB, BS, FRCS, 01590 623 226 /a/p/s 020 8731 7021, www.latimer-sayer.co.uk, Highgate Private Hospital, 020 8341 4182, and The Belvedere Private Hospital, 020 8311 4464

LAGUDA, KARDY, 07860 468 222, www.solidsounduk.com

LEADBITTER, ROGER, Chef, Stringfellow's, 16–19 Upper St Martin's Lane, WC2H 9EF, 020 7240 5534, www.stringfellows.com

LEE, PETER, 10 Linden Gardens, Notting Hill, W2, 020 7221 1238

LEWIS, EVA 020 7602 6253

LLEWELLYN, DAI, Sir

MCDERMOTT, BILGI, MA, 020 7381 9407, 07747 876 294

MATTHEWS, MEG

MATTI, BASIM, MB, ChB, FRCS, 30 Harley Street, London, W1G 9PW, 020 7637 9595, www.bmplasticsurgery.com

MAYNARD-ATEM, LISA, 07745 544 418

MEYER, HEIDI, YOHM Limited, 33–34 Chiswell Street, London SW1Y 4SF, 0845 456 6398, www.yohm.co.uk

MOSIMANN, ANTON, OBE, Mosimann's Private Dining Club, 11B West Halkin Street, Belgravia, SW1X 8JL, 020 7235 9625, www.mosimann.com

NORGAARD, IDA, DC, MSc, SCC, Dr of Chiropractic (USA), 33 Thurloe Place, London SW7 2HQ, 020 7581 5671, www.fix-a-spine.co.uk

NOVELLI, JEAN-CHRISTOPHE, Auberge du Lac, Brocket Hall International Ltd, Welwyn, Herts. AL8 7XG, 01707 368 888

Novelli Academy, Crouchmoor Farm, Stony Lane, Tea Green, Luton LU2 8PS, 01582 454 070

Novelli in the City, London Capital Club, 14 Abchurch Lane, London EC4 7B, 020 7717 0088

O'MAHONY, MALTI, Sister, Boston Clinics, 41 and 63a Moscow Road, Bayswater, W2 4JS, 020 7221 3904, www.boston-clinic.co.uk

PAGANO, ALBERTO, Ristorante Cappuccetto, 8/9 Moor Street, London W1, 020 7437 9472 www.alcappuccetto.co.uk

RETTER, NICK, Energise!, Hammersmith College, West London, 020 8748 9933, www.energizefitness.co.uk

RENSHAW, DANIELLE, 07855 958 682, www.ivoventuri.com

ROBSON-LAWRENCE, DEBRA, 144 Harley Street, London, W1G 7LE, 0845 230 2021, www.permanent-makeup.com

ROWLAND, STEVE, Family Dog Productions Ltd, www.steverowland-action.com

SHEIKH, RAHAT AFZAL, MBIH, EHP, NLP, Relaxation Response Medical Centre, 1 Harley Street, London W1G 9QA, 020 7838 0765, www.positivepeace.co.uk

SIMONER, RUPERT, Kempinski Grand Hotel des Bains, 7500 St Moritz, Switzerland, 0041 81838 3838

SADHURAM, NARI, Human Nature, 13 Malvern Road, London, NW6 5PS, 020 7328 5452

SALEH, ROY, Dr, MBChB, The Medispa Clinic, London Road, Adlington, Cheshire, SK104 4DU, 0845 605 6005

SANNA, PAOLO, Hair and Beauty Variations, Fortnum & Mason, 181 Piccadilly, W1A 1ER, 020 7437 3424

SHAUKAT, SIDRA, www.sidrashaukat.biz

SILVESTRY, LYDIA, www.lydiasilvestry.com

SINGH, RANI (representation: acting): Jaffrey Kent Management: 01753 785 162, (writing and presenting): Curtis Brown: 020 7393 4400

STRINGFELLOW, PETER, Stringfellow's, 16/19 Upper St Martin's Lane, WC2H 9EF, 020 7240 5534, www.stringfellows.com

STRIGNER, ANDREW, Dr, MB, BS, MFHom, 25 Devonshire Place, London W1G 6JD, 020 7935 4543, Fax 020 7935 5766

THOMAS, Alun, Holmes Place/Fulham, Normand Park, Lillie Road, SW6 7ST, 020 7471 0450

THOMAS, David, Holmes Place/Fulham, Normand Park, Lillie Road, SW6 7ST, 020 7471 0450

TURNER, BRIAN, CBE, Brian Turner Mayfair, Millennium Hotel, Grosvenor Square, London W1K 2HP, 020 7596 3444

TYMPANIDIS, PENELOPE, Dr, Renascence, 19 Wimpole Street, London W1G 8GE, 020 7462 0030, www.renascence.co.uk

TYRONE, Tyrone & Co, 14 Porchester Place, Marble Arch, W2 2BF, 020 7723 4843

UPPAL, RAKESH, BSc, MBCHB, FRCS, FRCS (C/Th), 149 Harley Street, London, W1G 6DE, 020 7935 6397, www.thelondonclinic.co.uk, r.uppal@thelondonclinic.co.uk

VANESSA, Vanessa's Hair and Beauty, 201 North End Road, West Kensington, W14 9NL, 020 7385 3674

VON SAXE, TATIANA

WARD, NEIL, Proprietor, Hair and Beauty Variations, Fortnum & Mason, 181 Piccadilly, W1A 1ER, 020 7437 3424

WEST, DAVID, Hey Jo Nightclub, 91 Jermyn Street, St James's, W1, 020 7930 3222, Eastenders Prime Wines, 020 7930 5272

WHITE, MARCO-PIERRE, Frankie's Italian Bar & Grill, 3 Yeoman's Row, Knightsbridge, SW3 2AL, 020 7590 9999

WILSON, VICTORIA, MInstChPLCh of Beauchamp Foot & Body Care, 41 Beauchamp Place, London SW3 1NX, 020 7225 0794

WOOD, TESSA, AGSM, PGDVS-CSSD, Dip Ed, TessaRossWood@aol.com

INDEX

A

Absolutely Fabulous 100
Accuvision 93, 95
    a patient's experience with Accuvision 94
    Wavefront Guided LASIK at
      Accuvision 95
acne 60
actinic ageing/skin cancer 61
acupressure 63, 66, 85
acupuncture 40, 85
addiction 14, 15, 16, 38, 85, 106, 122, 123
Adler, Larry 29
advice on cosmetic surgery 91
aerobics 35
    Laguda, Kardy 36
Afro-Caribbean beauty 55
ageing 21
Agent Provocateur 125
air fresheners
    aerosol 50
    Ecco Mist 50
    incense 50
alcohol
    alcoholic drinks 14
    dependency/addiction 15
alcohol and hypnotherapy 15
Alexander Technique 45, 85
allergy clinic 85
alternative health treatments 84
Anderton, Sophie 84
Antarctilyne 59
anthroscopic medicine 85
anti-ageing 22, 82
anti-ageing/rejuvenation 62
Anything You Can Cook 27
aphrodisiac 116
appendix, the 38
Aquamid 81
Armani 99
aromatherapy 85
arthritis 17, 37, 38, 120
Arton-Powell, Dave 43
Asian skin 56
aura-soma colour 85
Austin, Valerie 3, 15, 16, 109, 124, 125
    Austin technique 3
    Hypnosex 124, 125
    hypnotherapy for insomnia 109
    hypnotherapy for people who sleep near
      people who snore 108
    sexercises 124
    weight & hypnosis 4
autism integrated approach 85

Axt, Professor 35
    On the Joy of Laziness 35
Ayurveda 63, 85, 86
    Ayurveda Centre 75

B

back pain 43
    disc problems 44
    faulty movement patterns 44
    joint dysfunction 43
    muscle imbalance 44
    physical examination 44
    poor posture 44
back pain treatment
    muscle relaxation/stimulation 44
    rehabilitative exercises 44
    respiration 44
    spinal manipulation 44
    stabilisation/sensorimotor training 44
    workplace (ergonomic) and lifestyle
      advice 45
Balenciaga 49
ballroom dancing 36
bananas
    banana facts that may surprise you 3
    instant face lift 2
    many uses 2
Barbie 74
Baxendale, Dr Ronald 69
Beauchamp Foot & Body Care 48
beauty 53, 59, 79, 87
    Afro-Caribbean 55
    Asian 56
    beauty tips
    instant face lift 2
beauty treatments, home 66
    create your own spa at home 67
    exfoliating 67
    face masks 67
    hair treatments 68
    steaming 67
Beckham, David 110
Beckham, Victoria 2
belly dancing 36
    Chapman, Jacqueline 37
    health aspects 37
    mirage method 37
Belvedere Private Hospital 87
Berbatovci, Carlo 51, 52
Berry, Cicely 111
    Your Voice and How to Use It 111
Best, Angela 22
Best, Callum 22

Best, George 22
Beyond 100
Bi-Aura Stress Buster 75
Bibeveric, Nicholas 115
Bicom Resonance 85
bio-energy healing 85
Bird, Heather 22
Black, Sharon 58
black beauty 55
Blahnik, Manolo 85
Blair, Cherie 99
Blanchett, Cate 98
Blemishfree 59
Blood 38
Bloom, Adele 99
Bobbi Brown 53, 55
Bocaccio, Andrea 105
body conditioning 35
body lotions 50
body shapes 98, 99
Body Shop, The 113
Boots 50, 53, 54, 59, 60, 78
    Boots' "Muffles" 104, 108
    Boots' Shapers 2
Borissov, Valentin 15
Boston Clinics, The 33
    Boston Aesthetics Clinic 31, 80
    Boston Clinic 31, 84
    Boston Optimum Health Clinic 84
    O'Mahony, Sister Malti 31–32, 80
Botox 79
    all about Botox 81
Botox and other beauty procedures 79
    chemical peels 79
    collagen 79
    dermabrasion 79
    lunchtime peels 80
    skin lasers 79
    soft-tissue facial implants 80
Bourjois 54
Bowen, Mr Michael 20, 23, 26, 83, 117
    gynaecological and obstetric advice 117
    Titan Procedure 83
Bowen massage technique 69
Bowler, Dr Patrick 31, 33, 59, 83
    Intense Pulsed Light Treatment 83
    Tri-active 33
brain, the 27
breast enhancement, natural 85
Brewer, Liz 70
Brise 40
British Voice Association (BVA) 111
Brocklebank, Dr Anna, Lady 120, 122
    sex addiction 122

sexually transmitted diseases 120
bromelain 17
Bronze Tallulah 78
Brosi, Henry 6, 7
Brosnan, Pierce 86
bruises 17
Bruni, Georgina 2, 41
    Club 2000 2
    instant face lift 2
    morning energy boost 41
Buff's IncrEdible Edibles 30, 55
Bulgari 49
Bush, Gareth 6

C

C.A.C.I. 85
Cadell, Dr Ava 125
    Master Sexpert 125
Café Delancey 51
calcium 16, 38
Calvin Klein 49
Cancer Support Clinic 85
Capital Hotel 27
Capponi, Allessandra 86
Caprice 70, 71
Carter, Billy 58
cellulite 30, 32, 34
cellulite treatments and practitioners 31
    Boston Aesthetics Clinic 31
    Boston Clinic 31
    Bowler, Dr Patrick 33
    Endermologie 31
    Glancey, Dr Lucy 31
    Meso-Mesh 31
    Mesotherapy 31
    O'Mahony, Sister Malti 31
    Tri-active 33
Central School of Speech and Drama 111
Cetuem 54, 114
chakra balancing 85
Chanel 49, 53, 54, 99
Chapman, Jacqueline 36, 37, 40
    belly babies: pre- and post-natal classes 40
    the health aspects of belly dancing 37
Charles, HRH The Prince of Wales 2, 100, 101
Charles Worthington 75
chemical peels 79
Chinese Herbal Medicine 85
chiropody/podiatry 48, 85
chiropractic 40, 43, 45, 85
chlamydia 120
cholesterol 14, 18, 20, 33, 41
Christie, Julie 91
City Lit, London 111
Claridge's 6, 27
Clarins 31, 49, 56, 59, 78
Clarke, Nicky 58

Clinic of Russian Institute of Kibernatical Medicine 20
Clinique 29, 50, 53, 54, 55, 59
Clinton, Bill 121
Club 2000 2
Coca-Cola 6
Coen, Carina 66
    Mercarina Private Clinic 66
coffee 27
cognitive behavioural therapy (CBT) 123
collagen 60, 62, 73, 79, 80, 81, 83, 89
Collins, Joan 99
colonic irrigation 84
colour conscious 54
Colour Me Beautiful 53, 99
Colour Me Confident 98, 99
Comfort, Dr Alex 112
    The Joy of Sex 112
condoms 119, 120, 121
Connery, Sean 75
coronary heart disease 19
cosmetic acupuncture 85
cosmetic surgery 87, 90
    advice on 91
    Cosmetic Surgery Secrets 87
Costelloe, Ann 75
Countess Zena 123
Cox, Peter 9
    eating "up" the evolutionary scale 9
    food combining 11
Cragg, Dawn 97, 124
cramp 34
Crooks E45 60
Curtain Exchange, The 101
Curtis, Patrick 70
Cutera 83
Cutera lasers 82
Cynosure lasers 82
Cynosure UK Ltd 33

D

D'Addetta, Donata 86
D'Addetta, Stefania 86
D'Arcy, Deborah 15
Daily Mail "Best Dressed" list 99
Dale-Eliashiv, Orna 46
    Feldenkrais Method 46
Daly, Barbara 54
dance
    ballroom dancing 36
    belly dancing 36
    danceworks 36
    Killick, Paul 36
    salsa dancing 40
    Sleep, Wayne 35
Danceworks 36
Davies, Kristin 99

Debenhams 54
de Carle, John 93, 94
    eyes and eye care 94
décolleté 58, 60, 78, 82, 89, 90, 114
    Hand and Décolleté Serum 114
deep tissue massage 85
de Freitas, Alzira 71
de Havilland, Terry 100
Deida Acero 101
Deka's Tri-active 33
Dempster, Nigel 75
dental advice 13
dependency/addiction, alcohol 15
depression 29
dermabrasion 79
dermatologists 60
Dettori, Frankie 8
diabetes 19, 20, 21, 35, 118
    stabilise blood sugar 35
Diana, Princess of Wales 53, 84, 110
diet 1–11, 12–13, 15, 16, 18–19, 22, 31–33, 34, 40–41, 43, 62, 63, 85, 92, 96, 101, 117–118
    diet, alternatives 9
    diet, Atkins 40
    diets, cleaning 85
Dietrich, Marlene 16
Dior 49, 50, 53, 54, 99
disease prevention 18
Dorchester Hotel, The 6, 7, 75, 86, 101
Douglas, Michael 122, 123
Dr Denese 50, 60, 114
dress for beautiful health 64
drink
    alcoholic 14
    drinks, carbonated 12
    fruit juice 12
    getting dead drunk and snoring 108
    ginger tea 17
    isotonic energy drink 41
    power juicer 12
    tonic water 34
    water 12
drugs 16
Drysdale, William 2
Duchess of Cornwall, HRH 69

E

ear care 104
    remedies & methods 104
ear coning 85
Eastenders 41, 55
Eastenders' Prime Wines 14
Ecco Bella 50
Ecco Mist 50
Ecole de Ski Internationale 40
Elizabeth Arden 49, 50

Elvin, Brenda 63
EMDR 85
Endermologie 31
endorphins 29, 34, 73
Energize! gym 34
energy healing 85
Estée Lauder 50, 53, 54, 59, 60, 115
Evans, Joanne 82
Evolence 80
exercise 34, 42
　　aerobic 36
　　belly babies: pre- and post-natal classes
　　　　with a difference 40
　　exercise, body 42
　　exercises, facial 42
　　exercise to keep your body young and
　　　　fit 35
　　working with weights 35
exercise tips
　　Regain Your Figure: Easy Exercises for
　　　　Expectant and New Mothers 6
Extreme Make Overs 60, 96
eyes 93
　　Accuvision 95
　　eye care 93
　　eyes and eye care 94
　　laser eye surgery 93

F

face 66
facelifting, a short history of 88
face lifts, non-surgical
　　Medispa 72
face products 53
facial aesthetic micro enhancement 97
Farmilo-Fiumano Art Gallery 96
fashion 99
fatty tissues 30, 31, 32
Feldenkrais, Dr Moshe 46
Feldenkrais Method 46, 47, 48
　　healing pains and injuries 46
Ferrall-Peevey, Laura 77
fetishism 122
fish 27
　　fish, oily 27
　　fish, smoked 27
　　three-course fish menu 28
fitness, cardiovascular 34
"flab jab" 33
Fleming, Dr Richard 19
　　Stop Inflammation Now! 19
Fonda, Jane 1
food 1
　　diet foods 2
　　food combining 11
　　food tips 1
　　organic 40

food treats 1
foot care 48, 78, 85, 113
Forever Living Products 60
Fortnum and Mason 69
fragrant 49
Frankie's 8
Freiberger, Mr Malcolm 13
　　looking after your teeth 13
Frost, Sadie 60
Frostrup, Mariella 60
frotteurism 122
Fulham 39, 40
Fulham Pools 39

G

G-Spot 125
Garraud 50
Gemelle Clinic 86
general medical screening 85
Genie Complete 69
genital warts 121
Gerasimovich, Dr Viktor 20
Gillies, Vanessa Ann 69
Ginnings, Janet 70
Giorgio of Beverly Hills 49
Glancey, Dr Lucy 22, 31, 87, 89
　　Endermologie 31
　　Isolagen and Thread Lifting Procedures 89
Gold Spot 115
Goldwell 58
　　Goldwell Trendline 58
Golightly, Bertie 100
gonorrhoea 120
Grafenberg, Dr Ernest 125
Grant, Doris 11
　　Food Combining for Health 11
Grasso, Rosa 49
Gucci 100
Guenedy, Essam 100
Guerlain 49, 50
Guided LASIK 95
Guinness, Lulu 112
Gulamali, Dr Shiraz 13
　　Tooth loss 14
gym 34, 35, 39, 40, 41, 43, 71, 75, 77
　　gym gloves 35
gynaecological and obstetric advice 117
　　labour and delivery 119
　　pregnancy 118
　　puberty 117
　　sex 119

H

hair 66
　　hair and beauty variations 69, 70
　　hair colour and styling 70

hair extensions 70
hair removal 69
hair treatments 68
　　heated rollers and tongs 70
Hale Clinic, The 6, 8, 84, 86
　　service for children 86
Hall, Jerry 110, 112
Halliwell, Geri 77
hands 35, 61, 71, 78, 82, 85, 90, 101, 112, 114
　　Hand and Décolleté Serum 34
Hansen, Sally 71
Harrison, Audrey 86
Harrods 1
Hart, Dr Richard 14, 15, 17, 20, 104
Hawaiian Tropic 77
Hay, Dr William 11
HBV 69
healing, alternative
　　arnica 17
　　ginger 17
　　thuja 17
health and fitness clubs 40
health farms. *See spas*
Healthy Eating and Common Sense 14
hearing & sound 104, 105, 110
Heathcote, Peregrine 96
Heindke, Glen 39
Henderson, Veronique 98, 99
　　Colour Me Beautiful 99
　　Colour Me Confident 99
Hepburn, Audrey 100
herbal medicine 85
Hermès 49
herpes 120, 122
Hewitt, Denise 125
Highgate Private Hospital 87
Hill, Al 39
　　Tennis 39
Hill, Katy 70
Hillbrunner, Polly 74
HIV AIDS 121
Holland & Barrett 6
Holmes Place 39, 40
　　Holmes Place, Fulham 93
home beauty treatments 67
Home Microdermabrasion Kit 114
homeopathy 40, 85
Hooley, Joan 55
　　black beauty 55
Hopi 104, 110
Hopley, Jill 6
Hoppen, Kelly 101
Hot Gossip UK 2, 8, 14, 17, 30, 41, 58, 72,
　　78, 104
How to Marry A Millionaire 58
HRT 22
Human Nature 112. *See also massage; See*
　　also Sadhuram, Nari

Hurley, Liz 2, 91
Hypnosex 124, 125
hypnotherapy 123
   alcohol and hypnotherapy 15
   Austin, Valerie 3, 15, 16, 109, 124, 125
   D'Arcy, Deborah 15
   hypnotherapy for insomnia 109
   hypnotherapy for people who sleep near
      people who snore 108

I

I.D. Bare Essentials 54
incense 50
Indian head massage 63, 75, 112
Infinite Dress, the 63
insomnia 108
instant face lift 2
Intense Pulsed Light Treatment 83
intestines 38
Ion, Mr Lucian 92
   photo imaging 92
Isolagen 87, 89
Isolagen and Thread Lifting Procedures 89
isotonic energy drink 41

J

J-Lo 49
Jackson, Cindy 74, 87
   Cosmetic Surgery Secrets 87
   Living Doll 87
Jackson, Michael 87
James, Cornelia 100
Janet Ginnings Salon, The 70, 71
   Rigenera 71
   the Bollywood wax 71
Jazzy Bindi 57
jewellery 96
Jimmy Choo Couture 100
Jin Shin Jyutsu 85
Johnson's 77
joint mobility 38
joints, the 37, 38, 43, 46, 85, 86
Jones, Barry 89
Jones, Bridget 1
Jones, Sally-Anne 125
Jordan 99
Joseph 50, 100
Joy of Sex, The 112
Jungian Psychotherapy 85
Jungle Bronze 78

K

Kahn, Dan 75
Kama Sutra 119
Kardy's Dance Aerobic Party 36
Karidis, Mr Alex 91

advice on cosmetic surgery 91
Keith, Normandie 72
Kempinski, San Lawrenz
   Ayurveda Centre 75
Kempinski International Hotels 74
Kidd, Jodie 60
Killick, Paul 36
   Strictly Come Dancing 36
Kinesiology 6
Kingscote, Terry 113
   neuro-muscular massage 113
   sports massage 113
Kleankeepers 101
Kohl 56
Kors, Michael 50
Kournikova, Anna 86

L

L'Oreal 53, 54
labour and delivery 119
Lagerfeld 49
Laguda, Kardy 36, 105
   Kardy's Dance Aerobic Party 36
   What is Aerobic Exercise 36
Lancôme 49, 50, 53, 54, 59, 76, 77, 78
La Perla 114
La Prairie 69
La Senza 114
laser eye surgery 93
Latimer-Sayer, Mr Edward 74, 88
   a short history of facelifting 88
Lawson, Nigella 51
Leadbitter, Roger 115
Lee, Peter 15
Lemonburst 18, 50
Lewis, Eva 72
   Monochrome Body And Soul 72
Lia Therapy 85
Life Fitness 34
Lipodissolve 33
Lipostabil 33
liposuction 33, 90
Liquid Perfection 97
Living Doll 87
Llewellyn, Sir Dai 105
Lloyd-Webber, Andrew 105
lomi lomi massage 85
London Marathon 41
Lopez, Jennifer 54
Loren, Sophia 6, 91, 99
   Sophia Loren's Recipes and Memories 6
Louis Mariette 100
love & romance 115
Love, Courtney 112
Lucozade 41
Ludde, Patrick 70
Lumley, Joanna 12, 110

lunchtime peels 80
lungs, the 38
Lush 113
lymph nodes 38

M

Mac 53, 54, 55
Madesil Pharmacy 17
Madonna 39, 54
Majors, Farrah Fawcett 58
make-up 40, 50, 53–58, 59–60, 63, 69, 72,
   93, 96–98, 115, 124
   Make-up tips 57
   Shu Uemura Blending Brush 20BL 56
Marigolds 101
Marks and Spencer 100
Masochism 122
massage 66, 112, 113
   Indian head massage 63, 75, 112
   Kingscote, Terry 113
   lomi lomi massage 85
   neuro-muscular massage 113
   Sadhuram, Nari 112
   sports massage 40, 113
   tuna massage 86
   what good is a massage? 112
Matthews, Meg 71
Matti, Mr Basim 89, 90
   cosmetic surgery 90
Mavala 71
Max Factor 53
MaxiTan 78
Maybelline 54
Maynard-Atem, Lisa 100, 101
   why one needs a stylist to look like a
      goddess 100
McDermott, Bilgi 29
McKeith, Dr Gillian 18
   food abundance 18
McKeown, Dr 16, 17
McPherson, Elle 70
medication 16
Medispa 72
   Medispa and the MFLL 73
   Medispa Midface Lipo Lift 72
meditation 38, 106
   effects of relaxation deepen meditation
      technique 107
   meditation method 107
   Sufi meditation 107
menopause 18, 19, 22, 23, 26, 108, 117
   hot flushes 23
   mood changes 23
   the menopause and HRT 23
   thinning of the bones or osteoporosis 23
   Transitions For Health Inc 26
   Emerita Menopause Solutions 26

menus
  menu for love, suggested 115
  no wheat no dairy menu 7–8
  three course fish menu 28
    three course fragrant menu 52, 102
    three course menu – presentation 101, 102
Mercarina 66
  Mercarina Private Clinic 66
Meso-Mesh 31, 32
Mesotherapy 31, 32
Meyer, Heidi 38, 39
  YOHM Limited 39
Meyers, Loraine 86
Michelin 27, 101
mind, the 27
mind purification 85
Monochrome Body And Soul 72
  Lewis, Eva 72
  Pro-Lift 72
morning energy boost 41
Morreall, John 29
Mosimann, Anton 101, 103
  Mosimann's Private Dining Club 101
  Mosimann Academy 101
Mugler, Thierry 49
muscles, the 38
  muscle imbalance 44
  muscle relaxation/stimulation 44
music 105
My Beauty Secrets 63
Mystic Tan 77

N

nails 16, 48, 71, 78, 113
  Indian kitchen manicure and pedicure 71
Natural Beauty 67
natural breast enhancement 85
natural care 64
  dress for beautiful health 64
  secrets for youthful hair 64
  secrets for youthful skin 64
  secrets to a healthy mind 65
natural secrets 41
natural way, the 42
naturopathy 85
Naughty Janet 114
nerves, the 38
Net Therapy 85
neuro-muscular massage 113
Newman's Own 4
Nivea 77
NLP 85, 86
Norgaard, Ida 43, 45
  back pain 43
  posture 45
Nouba 54
Novelli, Jean-Christophe 8, 9

Classic Pipérade 9
Novelli Academy 8
Novelli at Auberge du Lac 8
Novelli in the City 9
nutrition 1–3, 9–10, 14, 18, 20, 35, 40,
  85–86, 92

O

O'Mahony, Sister Malti 31–32, 80
  all about botox 81
  Aquamid 81
  Boston Aesthetics Clinic 31, 80
  Boston Clinic 31
  Evolence 80
  Meso-Mesh 31
O'Mara, Kate 26
obstetric advice 117
oil, Almond 63
oil, Rosemary 63
Olay Deep Pore Cleanser 55
Onassis, Jacqueline Kennedy 1
On the Joy of Laziness 35
OPI 54
Orangeburst 60
organic food 3, 4, 6, 10, 40
orthopaedic medicine 85
Osbourne, Sharon 92
osteopathy 43, 85
osteoporosis 23, 26, 37, 38, 40, 45
osteoporosis, prevention of 38
Oxyjet 71

P

Pagano, Alberto 27
  Ristorante Cappuccetto 27
Parveen 99
  Parveen Couture 100
Patel, Mac 17
  Parmay Pharmacy 17
Patou 49
Peach on the Hill 57
perfect pout 59
perfume
  how many to try at once 50
  non-synthetic eau de parfum 50
  scents, ambiguous 50
  scents, longest lasting 50
  scents, sophisticated and sexy 49
  scents, sweet floral 49
  scents, sweet young fragrances 49
  scents, unusual and truly memorable 50
  scents that smell good on every skin 49
periodontal disease therapy 85
permanent make-up 96
personality 37, 98, 107
Pett, Caz 72

Phantom of the Opera 105
Photo imaging 92
Photo Rejuvenation 82
Pierre Marcolini 125
Pilates 43, 45
Pitt, Brad 75
PMT 16
  calcium tablets 16
  oil of evening primrose 16
podiatry 40
polarity therapy 85
posture 45
  how to practise good posture 45
  poor posture 45
  posture breaks when sitting 46
Prada 100
pregnancy 118
Prince Philip, HRH The Duke of
  Edinburgh 86, 101
Priory, The 16
Pro-Lift 72
Prozac 29
psychics
  Borissov, Valentin 15
  Lee, Peter 15
psychotherapy 123
  integrative psychotherapy 29
  McDermott, Bilgi 29
  Jungian psychotherapy 85
puberty 117
Purelogicol 50, 60

Q

Queen, HM The 100

R

Radcliffe, Paula 41
Rainbow Food Activity Chart 18
Rakus, Dr Rita 31
recipes
  braised lamb shanks 52
  chilled melon soup with mint and
    raspberries 28
  fish
  brill on sweet peppers & garlic 28
  cushions of Whitby/local smoked salmon
    with cockle & parsley dressing 28
  good health broth 42
  green pea soup with mint 52
  lavender and vanilla pannacotta 102
  marinated salmon with Cornish
    crabmeat 102
  Novelli's classic pipérade 9
  poached chicken breast stuffed with baby
    leeks and trompette mushrooms 102
  poached exotic fruits with passion fruit

coulis and lychee yoghurt sorbet 8
poached strawberries 52
salad of English asparagus with summer
    leaves and truffle dressing 7
steamed fillet of turbot "duglere" with
    balsamic reduction and yellow pepper
    sauce 7
yellow pepper coulis 7
Redken 58
reflexology 40, 85
Regaine for Women 72
Regain Your Figure: Easy Exercises for
    Expectant and New Mothers 40
Regenerate Yourself Younger 34
Reger, Aliza 114
Reger, Janet 114, 125
rehab centres.
    Priory, The 16
    See also sex addiction, treatments
Reiki 85
Rejuvanessence 86
Relaxaderm 59
relaxation 4, 21, 29, 31, 37, 38, 42, 44,
    48, 57, 63, 66–69, 74–75, 84, 94, 104,
    105–107, 109, 113
Relaxation Response Medical Centre 106
Renascence 60
Renshaw, Danielle 57
    make-up tips 57
    RMK Cosmetics 57
repetitive strain injuries (RSI) 46
Retter, Nick 34
    Energize! gym 34
Revlon 49, 53, 54
Rigenera 71
Ristorante Cappuccetto 27
RMK Cosmetics 57
Roberts, Julia 91
Robinson, Ann 91
Robson-Lawrence, Debra 96
    Extreme Make Overs 96
Rochas 49
Rodenburg, Patsy 111
    The Right To Speak 111
Rolfing 86
Romance 115
Roubi El Roubi 77, 99, 101
Rowland, Steve 104, 106

S

Sadhuram, Nari 112
    Human Nature 112
    what good is a massage? 112
sadism 122
Saint-Hill 99
Saleh, Dr Roy 72
    Medispa and the MFLL 73

Medispa Midface Lipo Lift 72
Sally Hair and Beauty shops 78, 115
salt 2, 3, 4, 17, 34
Sanctuary, The 78
Sanna, Paolo 70
    Hair and Beauty Variations 70
Savoy Grill, The 27
scents. *See perfume*
Schiffer, Claudia 87, 91
scientific proof for preventing disease and
    ageing 34
secrets for youthful hair 64
secrets for youthful skin 64
secrets to a healthy mind 65
sensual pleasures of sight 96
sex 115, 119, 124
    Cadell, Dr Ava 125
    Master Sexpert 125
    exercises and techniques 124
    scrotum exercise 124
    sexercises 124
    tone up those sexual muscles 124
    vaginal exercise 124
    Hypnosex 124, 125
    sex addiction 122
    The Joy of Sex by Dr Alex Comfort 112
sex addiction 122
    fetishism 122
    frotteurism 122
    masochism 122
    sadism 122
    transvestism 122
sex addiction, treatments
    cognitive behavioural therapy (CBT) 123
    hypnotherapy 123
    psychotherapy 123
    rehabilitation units 123
    Sex and Love Addicts Anonymous 123
Sex and the City 99, 124
Sexpert, Master 125
sexually transmitted diseases 120
    chlamydia 120
    genital warts 121
    gonorrhoea 120
    herpes 120
    HIV AIDS 121
    STD clinic 121
    syphilis 121
Sharie-Marie 100
Sharpe, Tom 123
Shaukat, Sidra 20–21, 30, 34–35, 55, 67, 79
    Botox and other treatments 79
    Buff's IncrEdible Edibles 30, 55
    exercise to keep your body young and
        fit 35
    Natural Beauty 20, 30, 67
    prevent ageing, prevent diabetes 21
    Regenerate Yourself Younger 20, 34

Sheikh, Rahat Afzal 106
    Relaxation Response Medical Centre 106
shen therapy 86
Shepherd, Richard 27
shiatsu 40
shyness counselling 86
sight 53, 59, 66, 76, 79, 84, 87, 93, 96.
    See also eyes
Silver, Avril 114
Silvestry, Lydia 63, 64
    Infinite Dress, the 63
    My Beauty Secrets 63
    natural care 64
Simoner, Rupert 75
Simpson's In The Strand 27
Singh, Rani 41, 56, 63
    Asian skin 56
skiing and snowboarding 40
skin and skin care 1–2, 12, 14, 16, 22–24,
    27, 30–33, 34, 37, 38–39, 48, 49, 50, 51,
    53, 54–58, 59–63
    skin, dark 54, 55
skin care products 50, 59
skin conditions 61
    acne 60
    actinic ageing/skin cancer 61
    anti-ageing/rejuvenation 62
    vitiligo 62
    warts 61
Skin Doctors 59, 60, 78
    Jungle Bronze 78
skin lasers 79
Sleep, Wayne 35
Slim-Fast 2
smell 49
smell & food 51
Smith, Clare 71
smoking 16
snoring 108
    getting dead drunk and snoring 108
    snoring, hypnotherapy 108
Snowden, Lisa 60
soft-tissue facial implants 80
soft drinks and juice 12
Soma Centre, The 82
Soneji, Mahesh 17
soul, the 27
sound & music 105
spas 72, 74
    Champneys 12, 72
    create your own spa at home 67
    Forest Mere 12, 72
    Pett, Cas 72
    Grayshott 12, 72
    Henlow Grange 72
    Kempinski International Hotels 74
    Le Sport Hotel, St Lucia 74
    Medispa 72

Ragdale Hall 72
Shrublands 72
The Dorchester, London 75
Spears, Britney 54
spinal manipulation 44
spleen 38
sports massage 40, 113
sports physician 86
STD clinic 121
STDs. *See sexually transmitted diseases*
step classes 35
St Ives 59
Strauss 105
   Also Sprach Zarathustra 105
Streisand, Barbra 54
stress management 86
"Stress Soother" tape 106
Strictly Come Dancing 36
Strigner, Dr Andrew 14, 15, 18
   alcohol dependency/addiction 15
   Healthy Eating and Common Sense 14
Stringfellow, Peter 115, 116
   Stringfellow's Cabaret of Angels 115
strokes 3, 20, 23, 25
stroking & massage 112
St Tropez 40, 78
stylists 101
Sufi meditation 107
sun exposure 76
surgery, cosmetic 87
Swarovski 71
swimming 39
Syal, Meera 70
syphilis 121

T

tanning 77
Tanning Shop, The 77
tans, fake 76
Taylor, Pam 60
teeth
   looking after your teeth 13
   tooth loss 14
tennis 39
Tesco 54, 60
Thatcher, Baroness 110
The Luxury Channel 114
The Right to Speak 111
Theron, Charlize 54
things of beauty 96
This Morning 27
Thomas, Alun 40
Thomas, David 40
   some fitness and nutrition myths 40
thread lift 87, 89
thymus 38
Time Out 51

Titan procedure 83
tonic water 34
touch 112, 114, 115, 124
touchy feely 114
Trager 86
transvestism 122
Trendco 72
Tri-active 33
trichology 86
Trinny and Susannah 99
Trump, Ivana 70
tuna massage 86
Turner, Brian 27, 28
   Anything You Can Cook 27
   Brian Turner Mayfair 27
   Ready Steady Cook 27
   Turner's Grill 27
Tympanidis, Dr Penelope 60, 61
   Extreme Make Overs 60
   Renascence 60
   skin conditions 61
Tyrone 71, 72
Tyrone and Company 71

U

Ultimo 114
unique relaxation response and
   meditation 107
Uppal, Mr Rakesh 19
UVA and UVB resistant wraparound sun
   glasses 93

V

Valentino 99
Valentino, Rudolph 110
Val Thorens 40
Vanessa's Hair and Beauty 69
van Outen, Denise 110
Vaseline 56
Versace 49, 99
veruccas 17
Viagra 115
vitamins 16
   vitamin C 16
vitiligo 62, 97
voice, educating the 110
voice – does it matter? 111
voices 110
von Saxe, Tatiana 42
   the natural way 42

W

Ward, Neil 69
Warren-Hill, Sheila 100
warts 17, 61
water 12, 40–41

water sports 39
Wavefront Guided LASIK 95
waxing 71
Way, Eric 99
Waynettas 45
weight
   alternatives to diet 2
   too thin 5
   weight & hypnosis 4
   weight and dieting tips 3
   weight reduction 86
Welch, Raquel 70
West, David 20
   Eastenders' Prime Wines 14
   Hey Jo nightclub 14
West, Mae 125
Westenius, Ritva 100
Westwood, Vivienne 49
What to wear 99
Whey to Go 2
White, Marco-Pierre 8
wigs 72
Williams, Robbie 77
Wilson, Samantha 106
   "Stress Soother" tape 106
Wilson, Victoria 48
   Beauchamp Foot & Body Care 48
   foot care 48
Windsor, The Duchess of 1
Winner, Michael 72
Witherspoon, Reese 54
Wood, Tessa 110
workouts, cardio 35

X

Xango 17

Y

Yalda, Nahren 56, 57
   Peach on the Hill 57
Yoga 37
Yoga and YOHM 38
YOHM Limited 39
Your Voice and How to Use It 111
YSL 49, 53, 54, 57, 100
Yugoslavia, Princess Katarina of,
   (da Silva, Mrs Desmond) 2

Z

Zane, Billy 86
Zeta-Jones, Catherine 91, 98, 122, 123
Zit Zapper 60

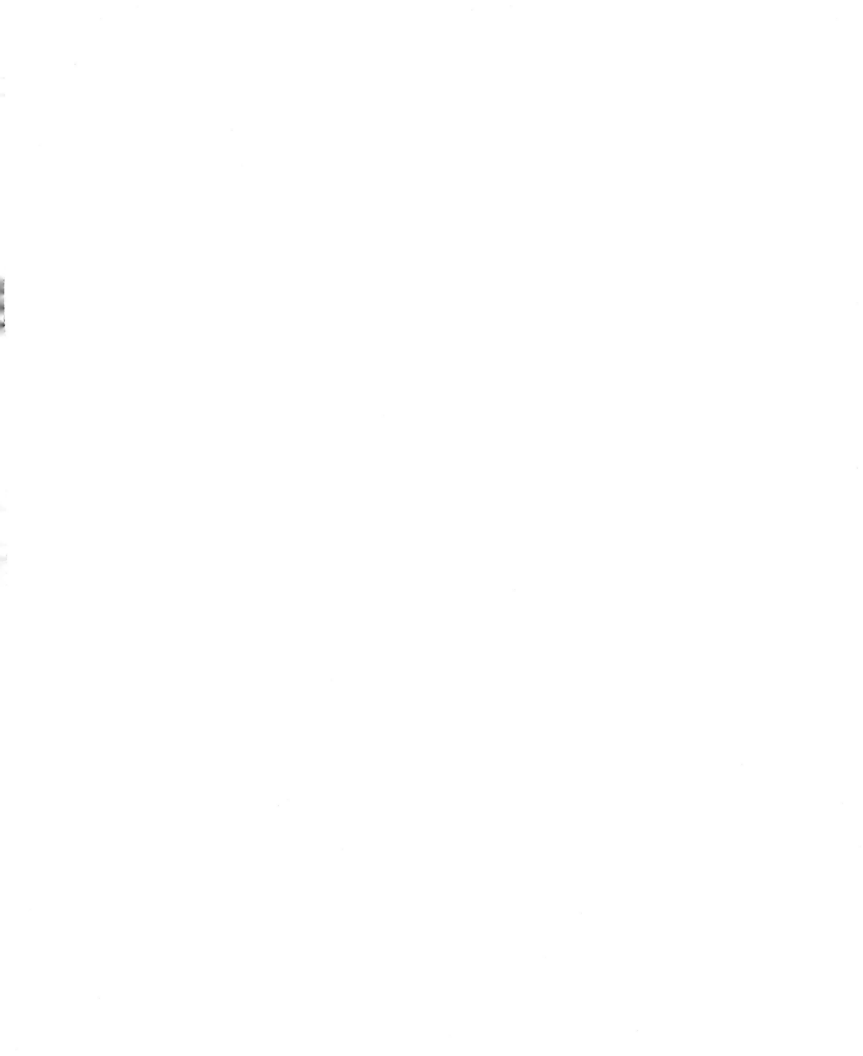